WITHDRAWN

CHIROPRACTIC

Consumer Health Library®
Series Editor: Stephen Barrett, M.D.
Technical Editor: Manfred Kroger, Ph.D.

Other titles in this series:

CHIROPRACTIC

THE VICTIM'S PERSPECTIVE

GEORGE MAGNER

EDITED BY
STEPHEN BARRETT, M.D.

WITH A FOREWORD BY
WILLIAM T. JARVIS, PH.D.

970167

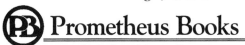

Prometheus Books

59 John Glenn Drive
Amherst, New York 14228-2197

Published in 1995 by Prometheus Books.

99 98 97 96 95   5   4   3   2   1

Library of Congress Cataloging-in-Publication Data

Magner, George .
    Chiropractic : The victim's perspective / George Magner : edited
by Stephen Barrett : foreword by William T. Jarvis
        p.   cm.
    Includes biographical references and index.
    ISBN 1-57392-041-X (hbk. : alk. paper)
    1. Chiropractic—Popular Works. 2. Chiropractors—Complications.
3. Chiropractic errors.   I. Barrett, Stephen 1933–
II. Jarvis, William T., 1935–   .   III Title
RZ242.M34   1995
615.5'34—dc20   95-21978
                                                          CIP

Printed in the United States on acid-free paper.

Contents

Foreword

William T. Jarvis, Ph.D.

I have studied the activities of chiropractors for nearly thirty years. I became interested while teaching health and physical education at a boarding school. As a gymnastics coach, I had noted that manipulative therapy seemed to help certain athletic injuries. In time, a neighborhood chiropractor began indoctrinating me. Although I had a master's degree in health education, my coursework had never covered chiropractic. I began reading everything I could find on the subject. The health-education literature was highly critical of chiropractic, but my mentor attributed this to prejudice. So I explored chiropractic literature to see what chiropractors said about themselves. What I saw convinced me that chiropractic was a cult whose participants were often victimized by their own misguided philosophy and training.

My doctoral dissertation, completed during the early 1970s, was based on a study assisted by nineteen chiropractors. My close association with these practitioners persuaded me that they were basically honest, hardworking, well-meaning individuals who believed that their treatment was effective even though no scientific studies had tested this belief. One of the chiropractors even acknowledged that the trouble with chiropractic was that it had never been proven scientifically. "What I do is treat patients the way I was taught," he said candidly. "Those who like it come back, those who don't like it do not. Enough people come back to keep me busy, so I must be helping them."

Many of these chiropractors proudly told me about patients who were almost miraculously relieved of their pain and dysfunction. When I asked whether they could tell which patients or conditions were likely to respond to their methods, all said they could not. How sad, I thought, that chiropractors had practiced for seventy-five years without determining what they can effectively do. Although nearly twenty-five more years have passed since that thought first occurred to me, chiropractic has still not made a single noteworthy contribution to the scientific knowledge of health care.

Chiropractic was founded on the delusion that spinal misalignments ("subluxations") have a profound effect upon bodily functions and that chiropractic "adjustments" may favorably alter these alleged conditions. Once this basic premise is accepted, it is easy to believe that nearly every patient will benefit from spinal manipulation. Chiropractic publications repeat and reinforce this mythology, distort scientific and government reports, and give credence to all sorts of pseudoscientific practices.

Many who choose chiropractic as a career have been misled by government policies and educational counseling materials that portray chiropractic as part of standard health care. Prospective students are lured by false promises of status and success. At most chiropractic colleges, students are exposed to cultlike indoctrination into a deviant belief system. They are taught false theories of disease and healing and persuaded to accept them as gospel. They are taught to disdain science and distrust medical doctors. A few reform-minded schools are trying to move away from teaching chiropractic philosophy as a substitute for science, but these are under attack as heretical.

Chiropractic students learn *conversational medicine*. This enables them to speak as if they know about disease and healing processes and creates the illusion that they understand medical science. Chiropractic literature, however, indicates that many chiropractors don't even understand the most basic concepts of disease etiology. Some chiropractic authors still attack the germ theory as erroneous, and speak of it as if it were scientific medicine's only theory of causation.

Many new graduates are dumped into the cold, hard world where survival values often displace ethics. Many discover that they are not in a true profession, but a guild of survivors who must sink or swim. A large percentage—half, according to chiropractic sources—fail in practice. This is one reason that chiropractors have the unhappy distinction of having the highest default rate of all who obtain Health Education Assistance Loans from the federal government. (Figures for 1994 showed that 1,547 chiropractors owed a total of $104 million.)

One chiropractor told me how he had gone from practice to practice trying to find a job that did not violate his conscience. Nearly every chiropractor who interviewed or hired him wanted high-volume work. In other words, "Just pop those spines and move on to the next patient." These chiropractors encouraged patients to return frequently for manipulations, a practice that can stretch ligaments, make joints less stable, and lead to more frequent musculoskeletal problems. My informant's greatest concern was the chiropractors who insisted that patients be x-rayed during nearly every visit. In an office where he worked, one woman had been x-rayed more than seventy times in a year-and-a-half. The idea of that much radiation exposure to a patient's body frightened him and caused him to quit the practice.

Chiropractic encourages self-delusion. One of the saddest stories I have encountered is that of a young chiropractic student with breast cancer who was so enthused over chiropractic's possibilities that she decided to make herself a documented test case. She died an agonizing death from untreated cancer but never lost faith in chiropractic's basic principles.

Chiropractic has failed the most fundamental scientific requirements that it define itself, determine its clinical usefulness and limitations, and conduct basic research on its mechanisms of action. Yet its public-relations spin-doctors attempt to portray chiropractic on an equal plane with scientific medicine by stating that both have their place. They maintain that both medicine and chiropractic have failings (and therefore the two are equal). These comparisons remind me of an experience I had as a boy while ice-skating in Minnesota. At the rink that I frequented, novices would skate around the edge while Olympians practiced in the middle. When an elite figure-skater fell while trying to do a triple Lutz, an old man who was shuffling around on his skates said with a twinkle, "I also fall down when I try to do a triple Lutz!"

From time to time, I am contacted by chiropractic students and practitioners who realize they have become ensnared by a deviant health-care system. By the time they see through the smoke and mirrors, they have invested a substantial amount of time and money in pursuit of their career. In addition, most rightly believe that manipulative therapy is useful. When they ask what they should do, I reply that there are two options: *run* or *fight*. By run, I mean get out of chiropractic and chalk up their losses to experience. By fight, I mean stay in chiropractic and try to transform it into a science-based service that focuses on manipulative therapy for musculoskeletal problems, mainly back pain. The more experience I garner, the more inclined I am to recommend running away. I do, however, salute and try to help those who become reformists and face the inevitable animosity of their colleagues.

George Magner has performed a valuable public service by looking critically at chiropractic mythology. Unlike most publications dealing with this subject, this book is comprehensive, extraordinarily well documented, and pulls no punches. Reading it might protect you from being victimized and could even save your life.

William T. Jarvis, Ph.D.
Professor of Health Promotion and
    Education
Loma Linda University
President, National Council Against
    Health Fraud, Inc.

About the Author

George J. Magner, III, received a bachelor of science degree *(magna cum laude)* in biology from Columbus College, Columbus, Georgia, in 1972 and spent a year as a graduate research assistant at Auburn University. He then worked for three years as a clinical laboratory technician and for eleven years as a biological research technician for the U.S. Department of Agriculture. In 1991, after concluding that chiropractors had permanently injured him, he founded Victims of Chiropractic, a support network and clearinghouse for information about chiropractic's hazards. Mr. Magner's royalties from the sale of this book have been donated to the National Council Against Health Fraud for use in public education.

About the Editor

Stephen Barrett, M.D., a retired psychiatrist, is a nationally renowned author, editor, and consumer advocate. He has been collecting information about chiropractic for more than twenty-five years. He is a board member of the National Council Against Health Fraud and chairs its Task Force on Victim Redress. His thirty-eight books include *The Health Robbers: A Close Look at Quackery in America; The Vitamin Pushers: How the "Health Food" Industry Is Selling America a Bill of Goods; Reader's Guide to "Alternative" Health Methods;* and four editions of the college textbook *Consumer Health: A Guide to Intelligent Decisions.*

Acknowledgments

I am grateful to the following individuals for their many helpful suggestions during the preparation of the manuscript:

Project manager   Mary A. Read, Assistant Editor
                                    Prometheus Books

Legal advisor   Michael Botts, Esq., Prescott, Wisconsin

Technical editor   Manfred Kroger, Ph.D.,
                                    Professor of Food Science
                                    The Pennsylvania State University

Consultants   Charles E. DuVall, Jr., D.C., President
                                    National Association for
                                    Chiropractic Medicine
                                    William T. Jarvis, Ph.D., Professor of
                                    Health Promotion and Education
                                    Loma Linda University
                                    Jack Raso, M.S., R.D., Editor
                                    Nutrition Forum Newsletter

I also thank the many people who shared their experiences and provided documents and other information important to my research.

A Note about References

Throughout this work, the numbers within brackets [ ] refer to references listed in Appendix C. The first page of a cited passage from a book may be indicated by a number after a colon, e.g., [23:57].

1

How I Became Involved

Why would I want to write critically about chiropractic? After I authored a newspaper article warning about the serious risks of chiropractic and its pseudoscientific elements, that is exactly what Thomas Kirchhofer, D.C., president of the Georgia Chiropractic Association, asked in a letter to the editor. The answer is the same today as it was when my article was published: I don't want anyone else to suffer the needless injuries that I and thousands of others have endured at the hands of chiropractors, especially without knowledge of the risks involved. I know from personal experience plus extensive research that chiropractic poses serious dangers. I feel morally obligated to offer my warnings whether you heed them or not.

My Personal Experience

My involvement with chiropractic began seven years ago when I experienced unrelenting pain due to a problem in my left lower back. Two medical doctors and a physical therapist could not help me, except to the extent that I could tolerate nonsteroidal anti-inflammatory drugs—and that was only for a few weeks. In desperation, I went to a chiropractor. What followed was a nightmare of incompetence I will never forget. I still suffer from neck and shoulder pain produced by the chiropractor's treatment.

After making two x-ray films of my neck and reviewing one of the lower part of my back, the chiropractor claimed that I had "subluxations"

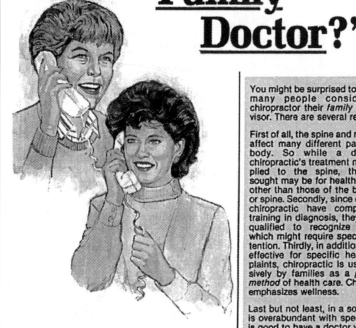

"So A Chiropractor Is Really A Family Doctor?"

You might be surprised to learn that many people consider their chiropractor their *family* health advisor. There are several reasons.

First of all, the spine and nerves can affect many different parts of the body. So while a doctor of chiropractic's treatment may be applied to the spine, the results sought may be for health problems other than those of the back, neck or spine. Secondly, since doctors of chiropractic have comprehensive training in diagnosis, they also are qualified to recognize problems which might require specialized attention. Thirdly, in addition to being effective for specific health complaints, chiropractic is used extensively by families as a *preventive method* of health care. Chiropractic emphasizes wellness.

Last but not least, in a society that is overabundant with specialists, it is good to have a doctor who looks at the human as a whole person. Chiropractors are reluctant to shuttle you from one specialist to another without good cause.

Are chiropractors a substitute for all other health-care practitioners? No, not at all. Some illnesses are complex and require specialized assistance. But your doctor of chiropractic is a good place to start.

Detach And Save This Important Health Information.

THIS ADVERTISING SUPPLEMENT IS PRESENTED BY AMERICA'S DOCTORS OF CHIROPRACTIC.

In 1988, the American Chiropractic Association, which represents about twenty thousand chiropractors, placed eight-page advertising inserts in two issues of the *Reader's Digest.* Almost every claim in the above message is either false or misleading.

in both areas. Although the pain was mainly in my back, he repeatedly "adjusted" (manipulated) my *neck*. The first five manipulations (one per visit) were uneventful, but the sixth was followed by new pain in the right side of the neck and across the top of the right shoulder, as well as continuous loud ringing in my ears, the medical term for which is tinnitus. I returned twice more to give the chiropractor a chance to try to correct the new problems. However, he didn't seem to have the slightest idea how to help me and even blamed my body by saying that my adjustments were "not holding."

To make a long story short, I consulted three other chiropractors during the next five months, for a total of eighteen more visits, four more x-rays, and about forty spinal manipulations. The tinnitus usually worsened after the adjustments, and a further complication developed after the eighth visit with the last chiropractor: I lost the full sensation of touch and felt tingling and "pins and needles" in the left side of my left foot.

I have consulted ear specialists about the tinnitus, a neurologist about the foot problem, and a general medical practitioner, an osteopathic physician, an orthopedist, and two physical therapists about the neck and shoulder pain; but there has been no improvement.

Why do I feel that I was treated improperly? In reading about my symptoms, I learned that manipulation of the neck can cause tinnitus by injuring arteries that supply blood to the ear. Yet the first chiropractor neither warned me about any complications nor accepted responsibility after I was injured. I also learned that manipulation of the neck is worthless as a treatment for back pain—which means that his treatment was completely inappropriate. The other chiropractors also failed to provide adequate warning.

Further Investigation

After thinking long and hard about what had happened, I resolved to learn as much as I could about chiropractors and what they do. Local public libraries provided some information, but the breakthrough I needed came after I learned about the National Council Against Health Fraud in an article in *The Reader's Digest*. I quickly telephoned and spoke with its president, William T. Jarvis, Ph.D., whose doctoral thesis involved a study of chiropractic. The fog of ignorance began to dissipate as he and others steered me to a wealth of eye-opening information on the subject.

Backed by my growing file of reliable information and encouraged by Dr. Jarvis, I decided to organize a group with two purposes. One would be to help people who believe they have been injured by a chiropractor. The other would be to help prevent such injuries through public education and a law requiring responsible informed consent.

Victims of Chiropractic (VOC) was set up in the spring of 1991, about two years after my final visit to a chiropractor. For a year, I placed ads every few weeks in *The Athens Observer*, offering free information to all who would send a stamped, self-addressed envelope. Many people responded. The newspaper article was published later that year. Following that, I began to put more effort into library research and writing. The VOC position paper titled "Can You Trust Your Chiropractor?" was completed in 1992 and published in 1994 in the book *Health Care in America: Opposing Viewpoints*. My continued research indicated that a more in-depth assessment of chiropractic was needed—hence this book.

My findings are important because reliable information can help people make choices in health care that they won't regret. My efforts may even help to change the health marketplace, which clearly tolerates deception and protects chiropractors rather than consumers. I have been privileged to share my findings with others investigating chiropractic, most notably Tim Smith, who wrote a powerful article on chiropractors and children in the *Wall Street Journal*, and with Rochelle Green of *Consumer Reports*, which published a landmark report in its June 1994 cover story. But VOC's primary activity has been to provide whatever support we can muster to the abused, suffering, confused, and emotionally distraught individuals who have been hurt by chiropractors.

Other Victims

Here are brief accounts of what happened to twenty people. Some came to my attention by telephoning for information and support. Information about the rest comes from accounts of legal actions and other well documented reports. Those identified by first name only (not their real name) either preferred anonymity or could not be reached to obtain permission to reveal their name.

- Mary Lehmann, a forty-four-year-old housewife and mother, enjoyed robust health but saw a chiropractor several times a year for minor back pain. In 1991, following manipulation of her neck, she suffered a stroke and became comatose in the chiropractor's office. Today she is unable to speak, requires help when she walks, and suffers from mental confusion. She is unable to swallow food and must be fed through a tube inserted into her stomach.

• Tina Frazier, a thirty-six-year-old accounting supervisor, had a stiff neck and went to a chiropractor. She ended up in the intensive care unit of the local hospital, suffering from a brainstem stroke. Her terrifying experience is described in Chapter 14. In a recent newspaper column, the chiropractor claimed that, through negligence, "M.D.s kill 5 times as many people as guns" and that he knew of no deaths due to chiropractic treatment in his state (Nevada) during the previous seventeen years.

• Bob, a forty-year-old college professor and former marathon runner, had his back "adjusted" regularly over a ten-year period. One tragic day, following manipulation of his neck, he became dizzy and collapsed, due to a stroke. Today he can barely walk or talk.

• Kristi A. Bedenbaugh, a former cheerleader and beauty queen, went to a chiropractor seeking relief from the pain of sinus headaches. During the second visit, she suffered a stroke immediately after the chiropractor manipulated her neck. She died three days later, one day before her twenty-fifth birthday. The autopsy revealed that the manipulation had split the inside walls of both of her vertebral arteries, causing blockage of the blood supply to the lower part of her brain. Chapter 14 discusses this type of complication.

• Karen Bell, while in her twenties, went to a chiropractor for neck pain and stiffness. Unknown to her, she had a four-inch-long tumor along her cervical spine. When the chiropractor manipulated her neck, the tumor ruptured, causing immediate paralysis. The tumor, which was benign, could have been removed safely and easily by a surgeon. But neither this chiropractor nor four others she had previously consulted had detected its presence. Karen now faces life paralyzed from the neck down.

• Tamara Joerns, a twenty-seven-year-old homemaker and mother of three, consulted a chiropractor for neck pain. Immediately after manipulation of her neck she became permanently paralyzed from the neck down and unable to speak.

- Julie Richers, during her early thirties, was active as a mother, 4-H club leader, and riding instructor before she suffered a stroke affecting one side of her body as a result of chiropractic neck manipulation. The disability is permanent. She states that she was never informed by the chiropractor of any possibility that this could happen.

- Margie, a forty-two-year-old designer, went to a chiropractor several years ago for treatment of pain in her feet and ankles. After that therapy, inexplicably, and despite her protest, he examined her neck and manipulated it vigorously. She awoke in the middle of the night with pains in her jaw, neck, shoulders, arms, and hands, most of which still bother her.

- Lynne Cramton, age nine, and her four-year-old brother Dale II visited a chiropractor because their mother wanted help for their ichthyosis (a congenital disorder in which the skin is scaly and resembles that of a fish). Claiming that vitamins would strengthen the children's immune system, the chiropractor prescribed regimens that included huge daily doses of vitamin A. Both children developed vitamin A poisoning within a few months. Although their acute symptoms subsided after the vitamin A was stopped, Lynne wound up with one leg several inches shorter than the other and Dale with permanent damage to his liver and spleen.

- Gladys Jones, a forty-two-year-old waitress, went to a chiropractor for knee pain, which she had endured for several months. He did not x-ray her knee. After the third manipulation of her knee, she experienced disabling pain. Orthopedic surgery was required to repair the torn cartilage in her knee.

- Christy Lewis, a forty-six-year-old woman, developed mid-back pain subsequent to a fall on an icy sidewalk. After the fourth adjustment of her thoracic spine by a chiropractor, she suffered excruciating pain from what she thought was a "heavy pressured adjustment" to her mid-back. Doctors at the nearby hospital determined that the chiropractor had fractured one of her ribs due to excessive force.

- Michael Crawford woke up one morning with pain in the left side of his neck. During his second appointment with a chiropractor, a neck manipulation caused severe aggravation of the condition, with pain radiating down his left arm and into his fingers. He could not raise his head from the table and screamed for help. A myelogram (special x-ray examination of the spinal cord) done at the hospital revealed a massive disc rupture, and surgery was performed. Neck stiffness and some impairment of arm function persist.

• Cesar Asuncion, a twenty-one-year-old college student, died ten days after discontinuing medication for epilepsy because a chiropractor promised that chiropractic treatment would revitalize his nerve endings. The chiropractor, who claimed to have cured at least fifteen other epileptics, was convicted of involuntary manslaughter and practicing medicine without a license. He was sentenced to a year in jail and three years' probation.

• Joseph, a sixty-five-year-old man, required dialysis (treatment with an artificial kidney) several times a week after his kidneys became seriously impaired. After a year, however, he stopped his treatment because a chiropractor promised that spinal manipulation and heat applied to the abdomen would fix the problem. Within fifteen days he had accumulated a large amount of fluid in his lungs and legs and had a near-fatal level of potassium in his blood. Although his life was saved by emergency medical treatment, he did not fully recover his strength.

• Arthur Rand, age fifty-six, after an attack of severe chest pain, consulted a chiropractor who considered himself qualified as a "chiropractic cardiologist." After conducting a detailed examination, the chiropractor prescribed nutritional supplements, exercise, and a low-fat diet. After six weeks of this regimen, Arthur collapsed and later underwent successful triple bypass surgery for coronary artery blockages.

• Myra, a chiropractor, developed back pain during her student days, where she was "taught to mistrust and even hate medical doctors and never to use medication." For seventeen years, she endured frequent severe pain despite going to a large number of highly experienced chiropractors. With each failure, she felt ashamed and blamed herself that her "Innate" was not responding. She finally consulted a rheumatologist who discovered that she had a form of arthritis called ankylosing spondylitis. Although she still has pain, she finally knows what is wrong with her and is getting some relief with medical treatment. She feels victimized because her chiropractic training had "brainwashed" her to avoid medical care.

• Linda Rosa, R.N., now forty-six, was forced to see a chiropractor throughout twelve of her childhood years. This occurred because the chiropractor convinced her mother that without one to three treatments *per week,* Linda would become blind and a hunchback. The chiropractor impoverished Linda's family and caused her to suffer back and abdominal pain for years after she stopped seeing him. Her full story appears in Appendix A.

• Michael Dunn, D.C., who now practices chiropractic in association with an orthopedic surgeon in Florida, became disillusioned soon after he began attending chiropractic college. After openly challenging chiropractic dogma, he was verbally abused by students and faculty members and even threatened with expulsion if he continued to challenge the validity of classroom presentations. Although he managed to complete school and develop a successful practice, many others in his situation have not been able to do so.

• Betty was taken to magistrate's court by a chiropractor after she refused to pay his bill. She had been suffering from medically diagnosed deafness caused by loss of blood supply to the ear. After the chiropractor said he might help, she began treatment but realized this was a mistake. At the magistrate's hearing, Betty offered evidence that deafness is outside the scope of chiropractic and that literature distributed by the chiropractor had falsely suggested that he could treat more than a hundred conditions (including appendicitis, epilepsy, and leukemia!). But the magistrate said Betty was responsible for the bill because the chiropractor had merely done "what chiropractors do."

• Peter Reshetniak, of Denver, Colorado, illustrates yet another way that people can be victimized. He is responsible for sharing medical expenses for his son, who lives with his former wife. He does not wish to pay for visits to a chiropractor who uses a fancy galvanometer to detect "energy imbalances" in his son's "acupuncture meridians" and "balances" the boy's "energy flow" by tapping along the "meridians" with a spring-loaded mallet. If Peter doesn't pay, he risks having to defend his refusal in court.

Are cases like the above unusual? Was my experience a fluke? Are chiropractors well trained in diagnosis? Do most perform treatment in a rational and scientific manner? Let's begin our inquiry by looking at chiropractic's origins.

2

A Brief History
of Chiropractic

Spinal manipulation of one sort or another has been practiced for thousands of years. Many cultures have had folk healers who practiced "bonesetting" to set fractures, reduce dislocations, and restore mobility to injured or diseased joints. Other healers have attempted to treat disease by ceremoniously manipulating or popping the joints [107]. Physicians have also used manipulative techniques, though usually in more restricted and responsible ways. In ancient Greece, Hippocrates (460–377 BCE), the father of medicine, used spinal manipulation to replace dislocated vertebrae, as did Galen (130–200 CE). Hippocrates wrote at least three books dealing with his treatment of bones and joints.

Until the middle of the nineteenth century, when manipulation's popularity increased, there were sporadic reports on its use by both medical and nonmedical practitioners. In 1831, a group of doctors in Massachusetts wrote that they believed that disordered spinal nerves were the true seat of disease. J. Evans Riadore, a London physician who practiced manipulation, wrote in his *Treatise on Irritation of the Spinal Nerves* (1842) that "if an organ is deficiently supplied with nervous energy or blood, its function is decreased, and sooner or later its structure becomes endangered." In 1850, a Reverend Isaac Harrington of New York claimed to cure disease by manipulation. According to newspaper report, Harrington theorized that every organ in the body was magnetically connected with the spinal marrow and that a sensitive person could detect and rectify irregularity of any organ by passing his hand over the vertebrae [84:115].

Not long afterward, physiologist Claude Bernard concluded that the nervous system played a critical role in health and disease, a concept that had become fashionable in medical and quasimedical thought [84:186]. In 1864, E. Dailly wrote an encyclopedia article stating that "therapeutic manipulations are of value in the treatment of all organic systems, and indications for their use can be found in almost all chronic illnesses" [84:69]. In 1867, Sir James Paget warned of possible complications of manipulation but encouraged medical practitioners to imitate the good parts of the bonesetters' practices.

In 1874, Andrew Taylor Still, who had medical training and probably had read of these ideas, established osteopathy with claims that diseases were caused by mechanical interference with nerve and blood supply. Still disparaged the drug practices of his day and regarded surgery as a last resort. He claimed that cures could result from manipulation of "deranged, displaced bones, nerves, muscles—removing all obstructions—thereby setting the machinery of life moving" [240]. Rejected as a cultist by organized medicine, he founded the first osteopathic school in Kirksville, Missouri, in 1892 [87].

D.D. Palmer's "Historic Leap of Reason"

Daniel David ("D.D.") Palmer (1845–1913) was fully aware of the bonesetters' work. He had studied osteopathy, knew Andrew Still, and was well read in the medical literature prior to his establishment of chiropractic. In the preceding years, D.D. had worked as a grocer in Davenport, Iowa, but sidelined in phrenology (diagnosing by analyzing bumps on the head) and eventually practiced as a full-time "magnetic healer." Writing about the latter in a newspaper column, D.D.'s brother Thomas stated: "His cures are made by the use of his hands only. He treats the cause of disease and not the effects. . . . He actually cures tumors and cancers without . . . medicine" [255:54]. During this period, Palmer sought to locate dysfunctional organs by touch and to impart a "life force from his hands . . . into that dormant organ, thereby assisting it to throw off the unnatural condition" [182]. D.D. also claimed to remedy inflamed nerves, a power he later attributed to spinal manipulation. In his *Text-Book of the Science, Art and Philosophy of Chiropractic*, published in 1910 and also called *The Chiropractor's Adjuster*, Palmer described his "search for the cause of disease":

I was a magnetic healer for nine years previous to discovering the principles which comprise the method known as Chiropractic.

During this period much of what was necessary to complete the science was worked out. I had discovered that many diseases were associated with derangements of the stomach, kidneys and other organs. . . .

One question was always uppermost in my mind in my search for the cause of disease. I desired to know why one person was ailing and his associate, eating at the same table, working in the same shop, at the same bench, was not. Why? What difference was there in the two persons that caused one to have pneumonia, catarrh, typhoid or rheumatism, while his partner, similarly situated, escaped? Why? This question had worried thousands for centuries and was answered in September, 1895. [181:18]

Chiropractic dates its origin to September 18, 1895, when Palmer manipulated a spinal bone (vertebra) that seemed to be out of place. He wrote of the occasion:

Harvey Lillard, a janitor . . . where I had my office, had been so deaf for 17 years that he could not hear the racket of a wagon or the ticking of a watch. I made inquiry as to the cause of his deafness and was informed that when he was exerting himself in a cramped, stooping position, he felt something give way in his back and immediately became deaf. An examination showed a vertebra racked from its normal position. I reasoned that if that vertebra was replaced, the man's hearing should be restored. With this object in view, a half-hour's talk persuaded Mr. Lillard to allow me to replace it. I racked it into position by using the spinous process as a lever and soon the man could hear as before. . . .

Shortly after this relief from deafness, I had a case of heart trouble which was not improving. I examined the spine and found a displaced vertebra pressing against the nerves which innervate the heart. I adjusted the vertebra and gave immediate relief. . . . Then I began to reason if two diseases, so dissimilar as deafness and heart trouble, came from impingement, a pressure on nerves, were not other diseases due to a similar cause? Thus the science (knowledge) and art (adjusting) of Chiropractic were formed at that time. I then began a systematic investigation for the cause of all diseases and have been amply rewarded. [181:18]

Palmer referred to the "displaced vertebrae" as "luxations." Shortly after the turn of the century, one of his disciples began calling these alleged problem areas "subluxations." The term "subluxation" soon became central to chiropractic theory and is still used by chiropractors today—though not necessarily in the same way (see Chapter 3).

In 1910, Palmer wrote that "the principles of chiropractic never was [sic] a theory with me. The first adjustment demonstrated it to be a fact" [181:407]. That same year, during a court case, his son Bartlett Joshua ("B.J.") was questioned about the Lillard incident. "B.J." contended that chiropractors had discovered a second system of nerve paths "not recorded in any anatomy I know anything of" [155].

Fact or Folklore?

Whether chiropractic's founding took place in the manner described above is debatable. Palmer specified that the bone he adjusted was the fourth thoracic vertebra (abbreviated "T4" and also called the fourth dorsal vertebra). However, the nerves that enable hearing are confined to the skull and are not located near the spine. If manipulation of T4 could relieve deafness due to a physical cause, one would expect that by now there would have been hundreds, if not thousands, of documented cases where it has happened. Alas, the scientific literature contains only a handful, with none reliably documented. Even the fanciful chiropractic nerve charts used by many chiropractors show no connection between T4 and the ability to hear. Samuel Homola, D.C., a chiropractor who has criticized chiropractic's unscientific aspects for more than thirty years, has stated:

> Referring to . . . Harvey Lillard, it is significant to note that there has never been a similar case demonstrated—in spite of the fact that chiropractors are daily engaged in correcting "subluxations" that supposedly exist in the spine of everyone. . . .
>
> It is [also] difficult to believe that any spinal joint, misplaced for 17 years, could suddenly and easily be restored, with an immediate correction of all the difficulties it had caused, leaving no permanent disorder of the supposedly affected tissues—locally or remotely. A displacement in the spine severe enough to cause a "bump" on the back would, of necessity, have to be a rather severe dislocation and, consequently, a quite crippling injury. In addition, adhesions usually form around displaced joints after a matter of weeks, and, over a period of time, muscles, ligaments, and other tissues shorten to accommodate the change in the joints. Yet Palmer was supposed to have made the correction in one treatment! [107:111]

Noting that Lillard allegedly had answered when Palmer *talked* to him, Homola suggested that Lillard had been only partially deaf and that his "recovery" was due to the power of suggestion. Willard Carver, D.C., one of Palmer's closest early associates, reported that the deafness had been confined to Lillard's left ear [28] [40]. Homola has also noted how chiropractic literature had designated T4 as the place to look for the cause and correction of heart trouble. He reasons:

> It would seem that a "subluxation" in the spine of Harvey Lillard severe enough to cause a visible "bump" would surely have stricken him down with heart disease. Yet, supposedly, the nerves of hearing, remotely enclosed within the skull, were affected by the disorder, resulting in deafness which lasted for 17 healthy years.

Did D.D. Palmer cure his "heart trouble" patient of heart disease? He did not describe the case in any detail, thus making it even more doubtful than the Lillard case. Furthermore, it is clear that spinal nerves do not control the functioning of the heart muscle. (The most obvious evidence of this fact is the success of heart-transplant operations, during which all structures connecting the heart to its donor are severed before the heart is given to the recipient.) Nor does the scientific literature contain a single verifiable report of heart disease cured through manipulation. Giving Palmer the benefit of the doubt, it is possible that the patient had referred pain whereby the discomfort originated in the back but felt as though it came from the chest.

There are additional reasons to doubt Palmer's credibility. He also claimed to have cured insanity by manipulation of T4 [166:51] and wrote that in 1888 he had discovered that hemiplegia (paralysis of one lateral half of the body) could be relieved by adjusting T5, apparently forgetting that he hadn't discovered chiropractic until seven years afterward [181:38]. Moreover, there are several conflicting accounts of the Lillard case [255] [260].

One of these accounts appeared in an unpublished manuscript written by Willard Carver. According to him, D.D. had been treating Lillard with magnetic healing and studied his back over the course of a week before delivering a single sharp blow to the spine that "almost instantly unstopped" Lillard's ear. Carver also reported that D.D. was a spiritualist and had contended that "the spirit of Dr. Jim Atkinson, a physician, who had died fifty years before . . . had communicated to him just what was the matter with Lillard, and just exactly what to do and how to do it" [40]. In a book published in 1950, B.J. Palmer insisted that the restoration was achieved by pushing on a bump in Lillard's *neck* on three successive days:

> We saw him "treat" Harvey Lillard. We KNOW it was IN THE NECK—not fourth dorsal as he wrote in his book.
> Why did he "treat" Harvey's deafness IN THE NECK and SAY it was at the fourth dorsal? Answer is simple. Medical men said and emphasized it was dangerous to do anything IN THE NECK. To move those vertebrae was to cause fracture or dislocation and cause

complete paralysis or immediate death by crushing spinal cord. Father absorbed this fear, notwithstanding evidence of having restored Harvey's hearing. Rather than have his students "treat" the neck and kill people, and kill off his Chiropractic idea, he shied all work away from neck and down lower on back where it was safer. [179:61]

B.J. added that by 1910, D.D. came to believe that neck manipulation was not dangerous, but he chose not to correct his previous writings. Sociologist Walter I. Wardwell, Ph.D., has observed that "like most folklore, chiropractic's comes in several versions" [255:57].

Regardless of the details, D.D. Palmer believed that in 1895, he had made a great discovery. Emboldened by his readings, by a fellow spiritualist's prophecy that he would create a revolutionary method of healing [160:10], and by his own penchant for transforming shaky theory into axiomatic truth, Palmer developed his dogma. He originally declared that misalignments of the spinal vertebrae cause abnormal nerve tension ("tone") in the nearby nerves and that disturbed nerve tone causes 95 percent of all disease. A few years later, he combined his spiritualistic beliefs into a biotheology involving "Innate Intelligence" or "nerve energy." This, he said, flows throughout the nervous system and controls every bodily activity not under voluntary control, but is hindered by even slight spinal misalignments.

In 1896, with help from a local minister named Samuel H. Weed, Palmer coined the name *chiropractic* from Greek words meaning "done by hand" [181:12]. That same year, he incorporated his first school: Palmer's School of Magnetic Cure, which was renamed Palmer School and Cure in 1897 and the Palmer Infirmary and Chiropractic Institute in 1902. During 1906, Palmer was convicted of practicing medicine without a license and served twenty-three days in jail. After he was released, his son B.J. refused to give him access to school grounds. Unable to resolve their disagreement over control of the school property, father and son submitted their dispute to an arbitration committee [166:46]. B.J. wound up purchasing the school and renamed it the Palmer School and Infirmary of Chiropractic in 1907, which customarily was referred to as the Palmer School of Chiropractic.

After the sale, D.D. moved to Oklahoma and later Oregon where he started other chiropractic schools. In Portland, he was ousted when students became dissatisfied. In 1910, he charged the unscholarly B.J. with plagiarism and commented that several of B.J.'s books were "not worth the paper they have worse than wasted because of their erroneous teachings" [181:639, 981]. In 1913, D.D. returned to Davenport where the continuous friction between father and son heated up and B.J. was accused of injuring D.D. with his car during a chiropractic parade. Two months later, D.D. died of typhoid fever. It is uncertain whether D.D. was actually struck by B.J.'s car. Some believed he was, but it could not be proven in court. There certainly was no love lost between the two Palmers. Both were dogmatic, contentious, and egocentric. Neither could get along with anyone as an equal. Essentially, B.J. ousted his father from leadership.

Chiropractic's Developer

Without question, Bartlett Joshua Palmer (1882–1961) had a stressful childhood. In the 1910 case he testified that, at the age of eleven, he had been "kicked from home, forced to make my living" [238]. He spent years as a vagrant, living largely by hustling on the streets, and slept in dry-goods boxes, hotel kitchens, pool halls, and the like. He was permanently expelled from school in the seventh grade, did jail time for petty thievery, and was well acquainted with the red-light district of town. In the preface to one of B.J.'s books, a dean of Palmer College wrote, "The first twenty years of this boy's life were spent in being educated to hate people and everything they did or were connected with" [104].

Much of the time, B.J.'s relationship with his father and two stepmothers was inimical. B.J. treated some people kindly—for example, he helped paroled prisoners find work—but he had misanthropic traits. R.C. Schafer, D.C., a former director of public affairs for the American Chiropractic Association, has reported:

> As self-proclaimed "keeper of the flame," he was suffocating and ruthless to anyone who dared oppose him. Dissent was not tolerated at the school, in his businesses, or at home, according to his son, David. Yet this autocrat knew how to retain the blind loyalty of his disciples, which in his later years consisted of a fundamentalist minority. He was described as an eccentric, a hypocrite, a tyrant, and a genius.
>
> I remember him as a bigot and outlandishly vulgar person. At an early age, I lived for 18 months in an apartment ... directly across from the Palmer School of Chiropractic when my father was a student there in the late 1930s. One day I saw B.J. approach and spit in the face of two students who were walking on the sidewalk. . . . I could not understand this and asked my dad what could cause such behavior. I was told that B.J. vehemently hated Jews and so acted on occasion—yet he would accept their tuition. It was common knowledge that B.J. . . . openly supported Hitler in the 1930s. [214]

Like his father, B.J. was afflicted by megalomania. His book titles reveal his enormous ego: *The Subluxation Specific*; *The Adjustment Specific; An Exposition of the Cause of All Disease* (1934), *The Bigness of the Fellow Within* (1949), *Upside Down and Right Side Up With B.J., Including the Greatest Mystery of History* (1953), *Fame and Fortune and the Know-How and Show-How to Attain It* (1955), and *Palmer's Law of Life* (1958). He made many sweeping pronouncements about the nature of health, disease, and the human body. He reportedly declared, for example, "When I saw there was no use for a sympathetic nervous system, I threw it out, and then just had to put something better in its place, so I discovered Direct Mental Impulse" [181:800]. According to his father, B.J. likewise disposed of the cranial nerves [84:161]. His ignorance and ego also combined to discover a "duct of Palmer connecting the spleen with the stomach."

B.J. acquired his chiropractic diploma in 1902. During his pre-chiropractic years, he had worked with a mesmerist and in a circus. These experiences may have honed his natural gifts in the area of showmanship and salesmanship, qualities that would help him make chiropractic what it is today. His charismatic, inspirational, and outlandish personality attracted throngs of listeners wherever he went. He was an impressive speaker. Followers adored him. Once he took over the school from his father, students came and left commissioned with religious zeal to "administer the wonders of chiropractic" and save the world through chiropractic. For B.J. and his disciples, chiropractic was not only a profession, it was a way of life.

From the beginning, B.J. did everything possible to distance chiropractic from medicine and osteopathy. He wrote his own textbook and developed a unique jargon for the profession. He took his father's theory a step further from reality by proclaiming that spinal misalignments pinch nerves as they exit the spine between the vertebrae. Even D.D. knew this was anatomically impossible and severely criticized this idea. But B.J.'s views came to dominate the new profession. He greatly expanded chiropractic's metaphysical basis, which constituted a major part of chiropractic education. He constantly derided the medical profession, using slogans such as "M.D. = more dope—more death" [255:73].

B.J. and his school emphasized salesmanship. He described chiropractic as a "health serve-us" [180:43]. He advertised extensively, first through print and later through his own radio station. Not surprisingly, chiropractic grew under B.J.'s leadership. However, his autocratic style offended some faculty members, creating numerous defections and schisms. The major debacle of his career took place in 1924, when he announced that his newly discovered neurocalometer would pinpoint the location of "subluxations" by registering skin-temperature differences along the spine (see Chapter 7). To a packed audience at his school's annual homecoming, B.J. decreed that all chiropractors must not only use the device but lease it for an exorbitant fee. The best of his faculty left, and enrollment in his school declined precipitously.

In the early 1930s, B.J. declared to the chiropractic world that only the topmost spinal bones should be manipulated, and that the rest of the spine would "fall into place." Characteristically, he gave the technique an outlandish name: Hole-In-One (H.I.O.). As noted by Homola:

> This new theory was considered by many to be a "dirty trick" on the thousands of chiropractors graduated by Palmer in years past and who had been completely convinced that vertebrae out-of-place at different points in the spine caused certain diseases—that it was necessary to adjust those specific vertebrae in order to cure these diseases. . . . Palmer's new theory . . . meant that all chiropractors were giving the wrong treatment unless they took additional training in the "latest findings of chiropractic." Needless to say, the "new theory" brought back many postgraduate students and attracted many new students to the Palmer school.
>
> One of the strange contradictions surrounding the behavior of many chiropractors who claim miraculous cures and unbending faith in their particular treatment method lies in the apparent willingness of these practitioners to switch their treatment methods and adopt new theories. . . . This contradiction in behavior and claims is also evident in the activities of many present-day chiropractors who eagerly enroll in one technique course after the other and who claim supreme healing powers for each new technique they employ. [107:173]

According to Morris Fishbein, M.D., editor of the *Journal of the American Medical Association*, the Hoosier Chiropractors' Association reacted even more harshly. It condemned the neurocalometer as "merely an instrument . . . to enable the user to increase his charges, which increase in his income has been boasted about by many of the users" [78:112].

Investigative reporter Ralph Lee Smith has noted yet another dimension to B.J. Palmer's belief system:

> Although B.J. alleged in his public writings that chiropractic treatment would cure all disease, when he was ill he went to see medical doctors in Davenport. Among other things, these doctors discovered that B.J.'s own spine was about the worst possible

advertisement for the value of chiropractic treatment that could be imagined. When B.J. developed a urinary tract problem, his spine was X-rayed by a competent group of specialists. "He had the worst-looking spine of anyone you've ever seen," the doctor who supervised the X-rays told me. "It showed very advanced degenerative arthritis with marked curvature." [232:11]

Later B.J. developed cancer of the colon and received medical treatment for it, including surgery, but he died of the disease in 1961 at the age of seventy-nine.

"Straights" versus "Mixers"

Several of the earliest chiropractors branched off in various directions. The most notable was Willard Carver, the attorney who unsuccessfully defended D.D. Palmer in 1906 against the charge of practicing medicine without a license. Later that year, Carver became a chiropractor, opened his own school, and began advocating other modalities in addition to spinal manipulation. B.J. Palmer championed "straight" chiropractic, so called because it involved hands only. When others began adding methods, some of which (like physiotherapy) were used by medical doctors, B.J. derisively called them "mixers."

The philosophical differences between "straights" and "mixers" have persisted up to the present time, with mixers increasingly outnumbering straights. Straights still tend to espouse the doctrine that almost all health problems are caused by misaligned vertebrae ("subluxations") that can be corrected by spinal adjustment. Today's mixers acknowledge that factors such as germs and hormones play a role in disease, but they tend to regard mechanical disturbances of the nervous system as the underlying cause of lowered resistance to disease. In addition to spinal manipulation, mixers may use nutritional methods, herbal remedies, homeopathy remedies, and various types of physiotherapy (heat, cold, traction, exercise, massage, and ultrasound). Straights tend to disparage medical diagnosis, claiming that examination of the spine is the proper way for chiropractors to analyze their patients. Mixers are more likely to diagnose medical conditions in addition to spinal abnormalities, and to refer patients to medical practitioners for treatment. The distinction between the two groups is not clear-cut, however. Some whose philosophy would be considered "straight," for example, use physiotherapy techniques, and some who use a wide range of modalities still hold literal beliefs in subluxation theory [241].

The Drive for Licensure

Seeking legal protection as well as public recognition, chiropractors began pressing for laws under which they could become licensed. Ralph Lee Smith has noted:

> From its infancy, chiropractic looked to politics and licensing, not as a way of working with science but as a protection against science. [Chiropractors] succeeded in getting licensure laws through thirty-two of the nation's forty-eight rurally dominated state legislatures by 1925, almost before the modern era of health care and health legislation began. . . .
>
> From the early 1920s on, legislators who were aware of the conflict between chiropractic and science felt that they were in a dilemma because so many states had already licensed chiropractors. A possible way out, they thought, was to vote for the license law which would at least give the state the power to control and limit chiropractic practice. [232:158]

The first law was passed in Kansas in 1913, but the first license was issued two years later by Arkansas. In 1915, the Massachusetts Supreme Judicial Court ruled that medicine was "not confined to the administering of medical substances or the use of surgical or other instruments," but included "the prevention, cure and alleviation of disease, the repair of injury, or treatment of abnormal or unusual states of the body and their restoration to a healthful condition." This broad definition said, in effect, that all valid health care is within the sphere of medicine. The court rejected chiropractic's claim that it was a valid alternative to medical care and reasoned that biological truth is not dual and contradictory. (Doubtless, some chiropractors agreed with that, adding that their system was the only valid one and that medicine was the blind alley.)

Before chiropractic licensing laws were passed, thousands of chiropractors were prosecuted for practicing medicine without a license. This typically resulted in a small fine, but many served brief jail sentences. Faced with prosecution, some chiropractors abandoned their trade. Some moved their practice to more liberal states, while others tried to conceal what they did by pretending to practice "physiotherapy," which did not require a license. Many aroused public sympathy by characterizing themselves as "martyrs." By 1931, thirty-seven states had passed a licensing law, and by 1950, the number totaled forty-three. The last of the holdouts was Louisiana, which succumbed in 1974.

In many of the states, the chiropractors' biggest obstacle to licensure was their own factionalism, for the mixers and straights disagreed vehemently about the proper nature and scope of chiropractic practice. The faction that could generate the most political pressure generally prevailed. On one occasion, D.D. Palmer himself urged the governor of Minnesota to veto a licensing bill, because Palmer disliked its broadly defined (mixer) scope of practice. The infighting among chiropractors resulted in widely divergent laws. For example, Oregon is a "mixer" state, in which chiropractors are permitted to do minor surgery, perform hypnosis, deliver babies, and prescribe nutritional supplements. In neighboring Washington, a "straight" state, the licensing law permits none of these things and does not even allow chiropractors to do physiotherapy [141].

Basic Science Boards

Chiropractors wanted licensing laws that would permit regulation by chiropractic standards, not medical standards. However, some states required graduates of chiropractic schools to pass an examination written by a basic science board before they could take one administered by the chiropractic board. By 1959, twenty-four states established basic science boards to conduct such examinations, the same tests taken by applicants for medical and osteopathic licensure.

The theory behind these laws was that health-care professionals should be tested concerning their entire scope of practice, and since chiropractors claimed to be able to treat the gamut of disease, they should be tested in such subjects as physiology, pathology, chemistry, and in some cases bacteriology, toxicology, and medical diagnosis. The majority of chiropractic graduates could not pass these tests. Statistics reported by historian J. Stuart Moore indicate that between 1927 and 1953, about 86 percent of about 47,000 medical students passed the exams, while only 23 percent of about 2,500 chiropractors succeeded. Nebraska was noteworthy because no chiropractor was able to pass the exam between 1929 and 1950. Of course, many chiropractors who failed the basic science exam either moved to a state where it was not required or practiced anyway without a license.

Most of the profession viewed the science tests as hostile, but, remarkably, at least one chiropractic school president, W. Alfred Budden, D.C., of Western States Chiropractic College, strongly supported them as helpful to chiropractic's credibility. Despite the support of an enlightened minority who wanted to accept the challenge of full-scope testing, some science boards were restricted to the spine so chiropractors could pass them. Between 1967 and 1979, however, all of the basic science laws were repealed [190:191]. (Tests must still be passed in some of the basic sciences, but chiropractic students are no longer judged by medical standards.) Some observers believed that the basic science boards were the main reason that chiropractic educational standards were raised from their once abysmal condition. Though much improved, chiropractic education is still vastly inferior to medical or osteopathic education (see Chapter 4).

Chiropractic Organizations

The earliest chiropractic organizations were set up primarily to help defend chiropractors arrested for practicing medicine without a license. Later, they were helpful in passing state licensing laws, improving education, and enhancing public relations.

Chiropractic organizations have been formed around the straight/mixer dichotomy. The mixers' organization is called the American Chiropractic Association (ACA), which traces its beginning to the National Chiropractic Association of the early 1920s. The ACA, with about 17,000 chiropractors and about 6,000 students, is the largest chiropractic organization.

The International Chiropractors Association (ICA) traces its roots to 1926 when B. J. Palmer started the Chiropractic Health Bureau. The ICA is the largest organization of straights, today claiming about 6,600 members (including students). Attempts to merge the ACA and ICA have failed due largely to the contempt—reminiscent of B.J. Palmer—that straights have toward mixers. The Federation of Straight Chiropractors and Organizations (FSCO), composed of "super-straight" practitioners, was started in 1976 and has about 1,500 members, including students. The World Chiropractic Alliance, founded in 1989, promotes super-straight philosophy but describes itself as "not linked to only one segment of the profession." Its 3,200 membership figure includes students and laypersons. Some chiropractors belong to more than one of these groups.

The National Association for Chiropractic Medicine, a reformist group started in 1984, has about three hundred members (see Chapter 17). The figures suggest that about half of today's 49,000-or-so chiropractors belong to none of these groups and, therefore, that none of them can credibly represent the entire profession.

Cancer Sufferers Finding New Hope Through Recent Discoveries

Happy results on thousands of cancer patients treated at the Spears Chiropractic Sanitarium and Hospital, Denver, Colo., indicate that we have found the major causes of cancer. And, the new 2,150-bed cancer unit now under construction will probably make this the largest private hospital and cancer center in the world. Well-authenticated literature explaining our research findings and results in cancer, arthritis and rheumatism, polio, multiple sclerosis, cerebral palsy, heart and other diseases is yours for the asking. We believe the public is entitled to know the great strides we have made both in our research and treatment of the problem as well as other diseases.

Amazing Diagnostic Cancer Test Perfected

For many years, scientists all over the world have been desperately searching for a simple diagnostic test by which cancer and

What Causes Cancer?

While others have searched for a cause of cancer originating outside the body, we have sought the cause inside the body. While others contended that some germ or irritation was probably at fault, we felt that disturbed body functions were generally to blame. One of the most important of our discoveries was that cancers do not result from any one cause. Regardless of their type, they appear to have three or more causes. These we have found to be:

(1) Interference with nerve supply to the area affected;
(2) Body wastes — poisons — resulting from poor elimination from one or more of the eliminative organs;
(3) Wrong foods and food combinations, which cause vitamin imbalances and over-

THE GUARANTEE

If given time for maximum results, Spears Hospital guarantees a refund of treatment costs to all cancer patients accepted under this plan who do not receive a cure, arrestment, relief, prolongation of life or other satisfactory results.

seldom a separate and distinct disease. It is usually the end product of other diseases and often flourishes in combination with other diseases. The major problem in diagnosing early cancer lies in the difficulty in discovering where certain other organic, all such diseases should be recognized and treated accordingly, even in their earliest stages. We now know what these diseases are.

Cancer End Product of Inflammatory Diseases

The "itis" diseases which most frequently pass from mild or in-

During the 1950s, Spears Chiropractic Hospital advertised that its "new discoveries . . . have given chiropractic probably the most universally accurate diagnostic test and the most logical and successful preventive and relief weapons in existence" for fighting cancer. Its guarantee offered "a refund of treatment costs to all cancer patients accepted under this plan who do not receive a cure, arrestment, relief, prolongation of life or other satisfactory results." Its tabloid newspapers contained many testimonial claims concerning multiple sclerosis, cerebral palsy, polio, arthritis, and diabetes (even though Spears himself took insulin under medical supervision).

Inpatient Facilities

Throughout chiropractic's early history, some of its schools and individual practitioners operated an infirmary, clinic, sanitarium, "health home," or hospital for patients who required nursing care. Historian Russell Gibbons estimates that between World Wars I and II, there were as many as a hundred of these facilities [88]. By far the largest was the Spears Chiropractic Hospital, established in Denver by Leo L. Spears, D.C. (1894–1956), a 1921 Palmer graduate. Spears Hospital opened with 236 beds in 1943 and was expanded to nearly 600 beds in 1949 [204]. During the 1950s, it was promoted as "one of the world's largest, most famous and successful cancer research and treatment centers."

Leo Spears was involved in many lawsuits and other controversies related to the flamboyant claims that sent patients flocking to his facility. After a 1951 *Colliers* article called the hospital "a quack institution," Spears filed suit but lost [268]. In 1954, he sued the Denver Better Business Bureau, the Denver *Post*, the Colorado Medical Society, and more than eighty other parties, alleging that they had conspired to damage his business. During the proceedings, a *Post* reporter followed up on eighty-three cancer patients whose records had been given to him by Spears. The reporter discovered that sixty were known or strongly believed to be dead and sixteen others had been diagnosed (without a biopsy) only at Spears Hospital. Other evidence in the case showed that some patients whose testimonials appeared in Spears literature had died before they were published. Spears lost the case, and, in 1964, Colorado passed a law prohibiting chiropractors from treating cancer [232]. The hospital closed in 1984 after a gradual decline in revenues. The main factor, according to Wardwell, was refusal of insurance carriers to pay for nonmedical hospital treatment [255:137].

Inferior Schools, "Superior" Claims

It appears that more than four hundred chiropractic schools have existed, but fewer than two hundred have had a significant number of graduates [73]. The largest number operating at one time (in 1925) was eighty-two. In 1935, when about fifty schools remained, the National Chiropractic Association (NCA) created a committee on educational standards. Higher standards were certainly needed. Between 1912 and 1935, medical literature contained scathing denunciations based on observations of chiropractic schools and various materials published by chiropractors [35].

In 1941, the NCA adopted accreditation standards and appointed a director of education named John Nugent. During his twenty-year reign, Nugent visited most of the schools, urged the smaller ones to merge, and pressed for higher educational standards [255:142]. In 1947, the NCA

During the 1970s, Palmer College published about fifty pamphlets, most of which contained unsubstantiated claims. The kidney pamphlet said: "If you are suffering from kidney trouble, the logical course is to visit your chiropractor. He will examine your spine to see where the trouble exists. A chiropractic adjustment will have you feeling better in no time." The liver pamphlet contended that "chiropractic is the only science which seeks to find the basic cause producing the abnormally functioning liver."

STUDY THIS CHART CAREFULLY!...

The practice of CHIROPRACTIC is as broad as the nerve system often called "THE MASTER SYSTEM OF THE HUMAN BODY." This MASTER SYSTEM regulates and controls all other systems of the body including the circulatory system, the digestive system, the respiratory system, the muscular system, the reproductive system, the glandular system, lymphatic system and eliminative system, etc.

Take time to study this famous "Health Chart of Chiropractic," and you can understand how important YOUR SPINE is in the maintenance of your normal "natural" good health. A misaligned spinal vertebrae can cause disease in ANY PART OF THE BODY. Notice how the nerves go to and energize every organ, tissue and living cell of your body—arms, legs, abdomen, head, etc.

Every health problem has a cause and the cause must be found and corrected before you can get well. Pick up the telephone now and make an appointment with your Doctor of Chiropractic for a chiropractic spine and nerve test.

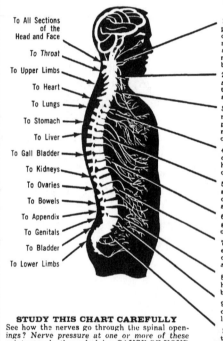

To All Sections
of the
Head and Face

To Throat

To Upper Limbs

To Heart

To Lungs

To Stomach

To Liver

To Gall Bladder

To Kidneys

To Ovaries

To Bowels

To Appendix

To Genitals

To Bladder

To Lower Limbs

STUDY THIS CHART CAREFULLY
See how the nerves go through the spinal openings? Nerve pressure at one or more of these points may be the underlying CAUSE OF YOUR CONDITION!

YOUR LIFELINE CHART

1. A slight "pinching" of nerves at this point can cause headaches, some eye diseases, ear problems, insomnia, abnormal blood pressure, colds, hay fever, sinus trouble, nervousness, wry or stiff neck, some types of arthritis, collic in babies, glandular trouble, etc.

2. A nerve difficulty in this part of the spine can be the cause of so-called throat trouble, neuralgia, pain in the shoulder and arms, goiter, nervous prostration, etc.

3. In this part of the spine, a "pinched" nerve can cause so-called bronchitis, *pain between the shoulder blades, rheumatism and neuritis of the arms, shoulder,* or hands, bursitis, etc.

4. A blocked nerve at this point can cause so-called nervous heart or fast heart, asthma, difficult breathing, bronchial congestion, etc.

5. Stomach and liver trouble, pleurisy and a score of other troubles, can be caused by pressure in this part of the spine.

6. Nerve pressure at this point can cause gall bladder problems, dyspepsia or gas of upper bowels, shingles, hiccups, etc.

7. Certain kidney problems or diseases, eruptions and other skin diseases can be caused by nerves being pinched in the spinal openings at this point.

8. Chiropractic adjustments here often helps such troubles as so-called lumbago, constipation, colitis, etc.

9. Nerve pressure at this point can cause bladder frequency, prostate problems, lower bowel and abdominal pains.

10. A slight slippage of one or both of the hip bones or the sacrum may cause so-called sciatica, leg or knee pains, and many other leg problems.

"Nerve charts" like this were commonly used during the 1960s and 1970s. This one claims that "pinched nerves" can cause bronchitis, gallbladder problems, goiter, liver and kidney trouble, and about fifty other diseases and conditions. It is inaccurate because: (1) very few of the conditions are amenable to chiropractic treatment, (2) the nervous system does not "control all other systems of the body," (3) the chart contains numerous anatomical errors and omissions, and (4) impingement of a nerve can cause such symptoms as pain, loss of sensation, muscle weakness, or paralysis, but it does not cause the diseases mentioned.

established a Council on Chiropractic Education, an accrediting agency that became autonomous in 1971 and gained recognition by the U.S. Office of Education in 1974 (see Chapter 4).

In 1961, the AMA launched a committee on quackery whose primary mission was to contain and eventually eliminate the chiropractic profession (see Chapter 11). Its activities were coordinated with those of the AMA's Department of Investigation, which collected and distributed information about questionable health practices. In 1966, the *Journal of the American Medical Association* published a devastating report on the educational background of chiropractic school faculties. The report was based on catalogs from each of the thirteen schools "approved" by chiropractic associations. Of the 267 faculty members named in the catalogs, only 126 (47 percent) were listed with recognized academic degrees, and twenty-three of these were not confirmed by the institutions alleged to have granted them. Only two individuals had Ph.D. degrees, one in anthropology and the other (whose holder was eighty-three years old) in chemistry. And many of those who taught basic science courses had no degree whatsoever in the subjects they taught [3].

Meanwhile, both in textbooks and in the marketplace, most chiropractors claimed that their treatment was superior to medical care and was appropriate for virtually the entire gamut of disease. The "meric system," developed during chiropractic's early years by B.J. Palmer and a colleague, was based on the notion that each joint of the spine can influence specific body structures and that "subluxations" of specific joints cause disease in their corresponding organs. The "nerve chart" shown on the opposite page is one of many that illustrate the meric system. Charts like these, as well as pamphlets published by Palmer College, chiropractic organizations, and many chiropractic supply houses, were abundant in chiropractic offices.

Questionable Ethics

During the 1960s and 1970s, chiropractic practice-building consultants became a conspicuous part of the chiropractic landscape [20] [22] [48]. Ads in chiropractic publications and frequent mailings to chiropractors offered courses and consultant services with claims of huge incomes and patient loads. One company, for example, boasted that its instructors saw several hundred patients per day. Another offered to teach chiropractors how to "build the $1,000,000 practice." Another taught "how to achieve the 'optimum gettable' with every patient." Many published testimonials or

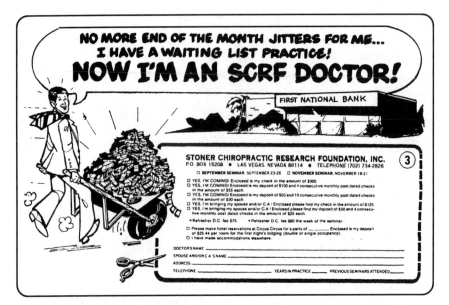

This portion of a two-page ad for a practice-building seminar from the September/October 1976 issue of *The Digest of Chiropractic Economics* depicts a smiling "doctor" wheeling money to his bank.

other notices stating how much money some of their clients were making. The most blatant financial pitch was probably the *Digest of Chiropractic Economics* ad depicting a chiropractor heading toward a bank with a wheelbarrow overflowing with money (see above). Although "practice-builders" covered some standard aspects of office-management, their main concern was how to attract new patients and keep them coming back (see Chapters 5 and 6).

The HEW Report

In 1968, the U.S. Department of Health, Education, and Welfare (HEW) published a comprehensive evaluation of chiropractic in the United States [53]. During the previous year, Congress had ordered the department to investigate whether Medicare coverage of nonmedical practitioners should be expanded. HEW's investigation, done with the help of forty-eight outside consultants, covered physical therapists, occupational therapists, clinical psychologists, social workers, speech pathologists, optometrists, audiologists, chiropractors, and naturopaths. In each case, professional

	Percent of Chiropractors Reporting	
TABLE 2	Treatment of Specified Conditions: 1963.	

Condition	Per-Cent	Condition	Per-Cent
Headache	98	Impaired Hearing	59
Sinusitis	94	Hemorrhoids	58
Constipation	94	Goiter	48
High blood pressure	93	Polio	47
Common cold	92	Diabetes mellitus	46
Asthma	89	Impaired vision	44
Bronchitis	86	Chorea	42
Low blood pressure	86	Rheumatic fever	37
Hay fever	83	Hepatitis	32
Gall bladder	82	Pneumonia	32
Colitis	80	Mumps	31
Diarrhea	79	Acute heart conditions	31
Ulcers	76	Appendicitis	30
Deficiency anemia	73	Pernicious anemia	24
Chronic heart condition	70	Cerebral hemorrhage	18
Genito-urinary	66	Lacerations	12
Mental, emotional	68	Fractures	9
Tonsillitis	67	Leukemia	8
Dermatitis	67	Cancer	7
Hives	60	Diphtheria	4

(The method of obtaining these diagnoses is unknown)

This table from the 1968 HEW report on chiropractic was based on a survey made in 1963 for the American Chiropractic Association.

organizations were asked to submit basic information about their professions, including: historical development; education and training; clinical and scientific basis of their practices; relationships with other health-care professionals; and needs of the elderly for their services. This information was provided both in writing and through direct testimony.

The expert review panel on chiropractic investigated thoroughly and quoted extensively from leading chiropractic textbooks and other current publications. The panelists noted that "since the philosophy of chiropractic is all-encompassing, its practitioners treat nearly every type of illness." The report included a table (shown above) based on a 1963 ACA survey in which 81 percent of respondents listed non-musculoskeletal problems among the three conditions they treated most often. The quoted statements included:

"The chiropractic way offers the safest, sanest, and most promising approach to the great majority of human ailments."

"Case records . . . demonstrate the effectiveness of Chiropractic with cases medically diagnosed as multiple sclerosis, encephalitis or sleeping sickness, hydrocephalus, epilepsy, sciatica, cirrhosis and cancer of the liver, and tumors."

"Experience has established the fact that . . . chiropractic adjusting is efficacious in handling both the acute and chronic cases of coronary occlusion."

"When the tonsils are slightly inflamed, . . . the doctor places the finger tip on the inflamed tonsil [and] strokes downward using a slight pressure . . . . determined by the tolerance of the patient."

"Tuberculosis is not contagious in adults."

The panel made an interesting speculation about why chiropractors and their patients develop mistaken beliefs related to curing disease:

The chiropractor attempts to move the vertebra with his hands so that it will not interfere with nerve function, It may be that . . . this maneuver is not affecting nerve function but actually is restoring the normal mobility of the joint. In this manner, the chiropractor may in many cases relieve pain and loss of function with the spinal adjustment. Referred pain to other parts of the body from joint dysfunction may be mistaken for a disease process, and when spinal adjustment relieves the pain, this may be thought to be a cure of the "disease."

Regarding chiropractic education, the panel noted the following shortcomings: "(1) lack of inpatient hospital training, (2) lack of adequately qualified faculty, (3) extremely low admission requirements for students, (4) lack of a nationally recognized accreditation body, and (5) such dissension within the profession that two separate accreditation programs must be maintained." The HEW report concluded:

• There is a body of basic scientific knowledge related to health, disease, and health care. Chiropractic practitioners ignore or take exception to much of this knowledge despite the fact that they have not undertaken adequate scientific research.

• There is no valid evidence that subluxation, if it exists, is a

During the 1970s, a leading chiropractic supplier marketed this message as an envelope or bumper sticker. It reflects chiropractic opposition to immunizations as well as to prescribed medications.

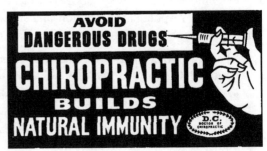

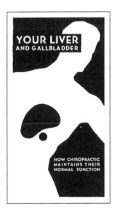

During the late 1960s and early 1970s, the American Chiropractic Association published many pamphlets containing flamboyant claims. This one stated that "there is but one method—chiropractic—that reaches directly to the cause of a malfunctioning liver or its associated gallbladder." The "Chiropractic Corrects Poliomyelitis " pamphlet claimed that the "foremost of the preventive measures is spinal hygiene" (periodic spinal examinations and adjustment). Other pamphlets advised: "If you do not enjoy good health, consult your chiropractor first."

significant factor in disease processes. Therefore, the broad application to health care of a diagnostic procedure such as spinal analysis and a treatment procedure such as spinal adjustment is not justified.

• The inadequacies of chiropractic education, coupled with a theory that de-emphasizes proven causative factors in disease processes, proven methods of treatment, and differential diagnosis, make it unlikely that a chiropractor can make an adequate diagnosis and know the appropriate treatment, and subsequently provide the indicated treatment or refer the patient. Lack of these capabilities in independent practitioners is undesirable because: appropriate treatment could be delayed or prevented entirely; appropriate treatment might be interrupted or stopped completely; the treatment offered could be contraindicated; all treatments have some risk involved with their administration, and inappropriate treatment exposes the patient to this risk unnecessarily.

• Manipulation (including chiropractic manipulation) may be a valuable technique for relief of pain due to loss of mobility of joints. Research in this area is inadequate; therefore, it is suggested that research that is based upon the scientific method be undertaken with respect to manipulation.

• Chiropractic theory and practice are not based upon the body of basic knowledge related to health, disease, and health care that has been widely accepted by the scientific community. Moreover, irrespective of its theory, the scope and quality of chiropractic education do not prepare the practitioner to make an adequate diagnosis and provide appropriate treatment. Therefore, it is recommended that chiropractic service not be covered in the Medicare program. [53]

Inching Ahead Nonetheless

Despite its obvious shortcomings, chiropractic was far from doomed. In the health marketplace, science is not all that counts. Politics and persistence are more important, and chiropractors have always excelled in these. During the 1970s, they achieved licensure in the remaining states, gained partial coverage under Medicare, gained increased coverage through other insurance plans, achieved recognition for their own accrediting agency, filed lawsuits that stopped organized medicine's antichiropractic campaign, and began making significant improvements in their educational system. During the past few years, chiropractic leaders have initiated efforts to curb unethical behavior, develop practice standards, and generate meaningful research, while the scientific community has acknowledged that spinal manipulation may be helpful in appropriately selected cases of low-back pain.

Does this mean that most chiropractors now practice in a scientific manner? Or that spinal manipulation by chiropractors is necessarily safe? Or that most people who consult a chiropractor are likely to be appropriately diagnosed and sensibly treated? In my opinion, the answer to each of these questions is still *no*.

Read on!

3

The Elusive
"Subluxation"

During the late 1970s, Dr. Stephen Barrett made the following observation in an editorial published in a medicolegal journal:

> To the average person, chiropractic can appear very attractive. Chiropractors are licensed as doctors. Their schools are being accredited. They are covered by Medicare and many other third-party carriers. Most of them are sincere and personable. But are they *doctors?* Can a house be built without a foundation? [17]

This chapter examines chiropractic's theoretical foundation.

What Do Chiropractors Believe?

Do most of today's chiropractors believe that too little or too much "nerve tone" is the cause of most disease? Or that "Innate Intelligence" or "nerve energy" flows throughout the nervous system and controls every bodily activity not under voluntary control, but is hindered by even slight spinal misalignments? Or that the cause of disease is misalignments that pinch the spinal nerves as they exit the spine between the vertebrae? Do chiropractors believe that "subluxations" are displaced bones that can be seen on x-rays and can be put back in place by spinal adjustments?

Although in 1975 the American Chiropractic Association (ACA) "disaffirmed the [monocausal] doctrine that holds to a singular approach to the treatment of disease," the ACA's current "Chiropractic: State of the Art" booklet states that "classical subluxation" theory and the "nerve compression hypothesis" still occupy a "central place in the chiropractic rationale" [46]. Recent brochures from the International Chiropractors Association (ICA) describe "subluxations" as misaligned vertebrae that "may cause . . . dysfunction in muscle, lymphatic, and organ tissue as well as imbalance in normal body processes" [72]. The ICA policy handbook states that "subluxation is a responsible and credible diagnosis" [195]. "Super-straight" chiropractors maintain that chiropractic's sole purpose is locating and correcting subluxations and that chiropractors neither diagnose nor treat disease.

In 1980, a prominent chiropractic educator asked one thousand chiropractors on the ACA's mailing list whether they agreed with various statements related to such beliefs [201]. Of 268 respondents, only twelve (4 percent) agreed that "the chiropractic subluxation" is "the cause of all disease," but 188 (70 percent) agreed that "the chiropractic subluxation may be related to the cause of most disease." When asked whether "the chiropractic monocausal theory is scientifically supported," twelve out of 260 (5 percent) said "completely," 195 (75 percent) said "partially," and 53 (20 percent) said "not at all." Only 37 (14 percent) checked "I do not believe that the chiropractic subluxation is a significant cause of disease." When asked to check off "the degree of importance you believe subluxation plays," 253 out of 268 (94 percent) checked "50%" or higher for musculoskeletal problems and 206 (78 percent) out of 265 checked "50%" or more for visceral disease problems (see charts opposite). Had members of the International Chiropractors Association or other "straight" chiropractic groups been asked the same questions, their responses would have shown greater degrees of belief in subluxation theory.

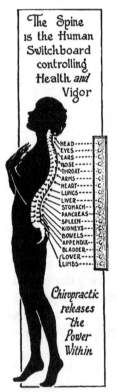

The Spine is the Human Switchboard controlling Health and Vigor

HEAD
EYES
EARS
NOSE
THROAT
ARMS
HEART
LUNGS
LIVER
STOMACH
PANCREAS
SPLEEN
KIDNEYS
BOWELS
APPENDIX
BLADDER
(LOWER
LIMBS

Chiropractic releases the Power Within

Source: *Spears Sanigram* #66, late 1960s.

Ponder for a moment what these answers mean. How can chiropractic's monocausal theory (the Palmerian notion that subluxations are the basic cause of disease) be "partially scientifically supported"? How can "subluxation" be "20% important," "50% important," "70% important," or "90% important" as a cause of disease? Do such answers reflect confusion, controversy, obfuscation—or some of each? Let's begin our inquiry by examining how the word "subluxation" has been defined.

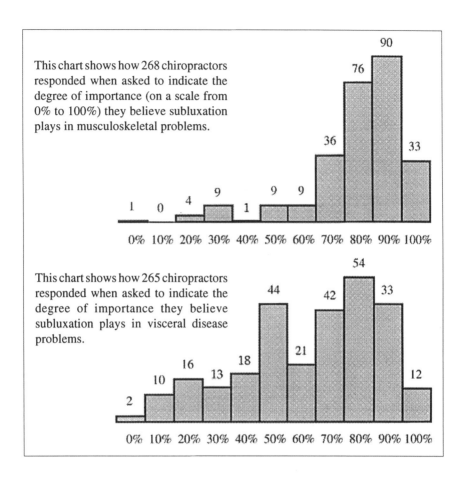

This chart shows how 268 chiropractors responded when asked to indicate the degree of importance (on a scale from 0% to 100%) they believe subluxation plays in musculoskeletal problems.

This chart shows how 265 chiropractors responded when asked to indicate the degree of importance they believe subluxation plays in visceral disease problems.

Subluxations: Real versus Imaginary

Medical doctors and chiropractors use the term "subluxation" differently. The medical meaning is incomplete or partial dislocation—a condition in which the bony surfaces of a joint no longer face each other exactly but remain in partial contact. However, most physicians use the term *partial dislocation* rather than subluxation. Most partial dislocations occur in areas other than the spine and are the result of injury. Since the ligaments attached to the spinal bones are extremely strong, dislocations are rare after birth and are unlikely to occur without severe injury that would require surgical treatment, not manipulation. There is a condition called *spondylolisthesis*, which is a slippage of a vertebra relative to another. This condition is usually present at birth, is visible on x-ray films, and commonly causes no symptoms.

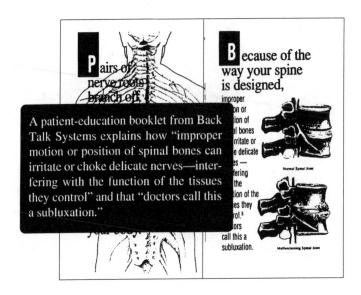

A patient-education booklet from Back Talk Systems explains how "improper motion or position of spinal bones can irritate or choke delicate nerves—interfering with the function of the tissues they control" and that "doctors call this a subluxation."

Chiropractors, on the other hand, do not agree on how the word "subluxation" should be defined [83] [143]. Some speak of "bones out of place" and/or "pinched nerves," some think in terms of "fixations" and/or decreased joint mobility, some occupy a middle ground in which any or all may play a role, and a few (as noted in Chapter 17) renounce chiropractic's subluxation concepts completely.

The most "modern" chiropractic definition was developed a few years ago by the Consortium for Chiropractic Research, a group led by chiropractic educators interested in research. They define subluxation as "a motion segment in which alignment, movement integrity and/or physiologic function are altered, although contact between the joint surfaces remains intact." Although presumably well intended, this definition is so broad that it enables chiropractors to apply the term "subluxation" to any condition, real or imaginary, they would like to treat.

Are Chiropractic Subluxations Visible?

In 1964, when asked to demonstrate that its subluxations actually show on x-ray films, chiropractic failed miserably. During the early 1960s, the National Association of Letter Carriers (NALC) included chiropractic in its health plan, with coverage limited to "spinal adjustments by hand for the treatment of vertebral subluxations or misalignments." In 1966, NALC's director of health insurance reported:

Almost from the inception of the program, we encountered trouble with chiropractic claims. Expenses were submitted for x-rays that could not be interpreted, due to the poor technical quality of the films; claims were made for the treatment of measles, mumps, heart trouble, mental retardation, female disorders and sundry other ailments. None of these conditions has any medical relationship to vertebral subluxations or spinal misalignments. . . .

The leaders of both the ACA and ICA made repeated efforts to impress upon their membership the gravity of the situation, and the need to halt and prevent further abuses of insurance benefits. For reasons I cannot explain, these efforts produced no discernible improvement. . . .

At our invitation, representatives of both the ACA and ICA met in our office with one of the most reputable radiologists in the area, whom we had engaged on a temporary consultant basis.

Our doctor (medical) presented 20 sets of x-rays that had been submitted by chiropractors. Each film was purported to show a subluxation; in several instances, four to six subluxations had been diagnosed in a single x-ray.

One after another, each film was placed in the view box. The chiropractic representatives, including a radiologist of their own selection, were invited to point out the subluxations. Not a single one was identified. Nor did the chiropractic representatives offer a solitary comment. [62]

In 1971, Dr. Barrett challenged a local chiropractic society to produce ten sets of "before and after" x-rays that demonstrate the effect of chiropractic treatment. The chiropractors refused and suggested that he contact

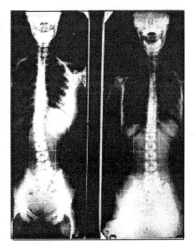

These "before and after x-rays" were included in a widely used chiropractic textbook as "proof" that chiropractic adjustments had been effective in correcting distortion of the spine of a twenty-year-old woman with "constipation, appendicitis in severe form" [149]. No details were given about the patient's history, physical exam, or laboratory findings. Both films were overexposed, obscuring most of the pelvis and almost all of the spine. The patient received two large doses of ionizing radiation to her sexual organs.

the Palmer School of Chiropractic to inspect some from its "teaching files." When he did, however, Palmer vice president Ronald Frogley, D.C., replied:

> Chiropractors do not make the claim to be able to read a specific subluxation from an x-ray film. [They] can read spinal distortion, which indicates the possible presence of a subluxation and can confirm the actual presence of a subluxation by other physical findings.

Despite all this, in 1972, Congress passed a law enabling chiropractors to collect from Medicare for "manual manipulation of the spine (to correct a subluxation demonstrated by x-ray to exist)" [234]. A few weeks after the law was passed, Doyl Taylor, head of the AMA Department of Investigation, told Barrett that when chiropractic inclusion appeared inevitable, the "subluxation" language was inserted with the hope of preventing chiropractors from actually being paid. The idea's originator thought that since chiropractic's traditional "subluxations" were visible only to chiropractors, this provision would sabotage their coverage. After the law was passed, however, two things happened to enable payment. First, chiropractors held a consensus conference that redefined "subluxations" to include common

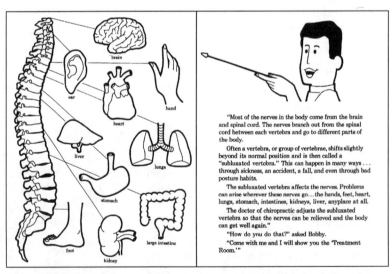

"Bobby and Sue Visit the Doctor of Chiropractic," a coloring storybook distributed by the ACA during most of the 1970s, states that "the subluxated vertebra affects the nerves," that "problems can arise wherever these nerves go," and that problems are fixed when "subluxated vertebrae are restored to their normal position" by chiropractic adjustments [113].

findings that others could see. Second, according to Taylor, the government officials responsible for interpreting the new law "decided that Congress intended chiropractors to be paid for something." The regulators then defined subluxation as "an incomplete dislocation, off-centering, misalignment, fixation, or abnormal spacing of the vertebrae" and stipulated that the "primary diagnosis" must be a subluxation.

The consensus conference, held in Houston in November 1972, resulted in the following statement:

> A *subluxation* is the alteration of the normal dynamics, anatomical or physiological relationships of contiguous articular structures. In evaluation of this complex phenomenon, we find that it has—or may have—biomechanical, pathophysiological, clinical, radiologic, and other manifestations. [211]

The document, several pages long, described the supposed radiologic manifestations of eighteen types of "subluxations," including "flexion malposition," "extension malposition," "lateral flexion malposition," "rotational malposition," "hypomobility" (also called "fixation subluxation"), "hypermobility," "aberrant motion," "altered interosseous spacing," "foraminal occlusion," scoliosis, and several conditions in which "gross displacements" are evident. Some are fancy names for the minor degenerative changes that occur as people age; they often have nothing to do with a patient's symptoms and are not changed by chiropractic treatment. Some, as acknowledged by the Houston conferees, are not even visible on x-ray films. Labeling them "subluxations" is simply a device to get paid. Since 1973, Medicare has paid more than two billion dollars for treating chiropractic "subluxations"!

Topflight academic chiropractors regard "subluxations" more realistically. In 1987, Williams & Wilkins, a prominent medical textbook publisher, issued "the most comprehensive chiropractic radiology text ever published!" Titled *Essentials of Skeletal Radiology,* the book was produced by professors who teach radiology at chiropractic colleges. It contains over three thousand illustrations and reads like a standard medical text [271]. When Barrett scanned it and inspected its index, he was unable to find a single mention of the word "subluxation."

An equally interesting observation was made during a recent interview of John J. Triano, D.C., a chiropractor with a degree in neurophysiology who teaches and conducts research at National College of Chiropractic. When an astute reporter asked whether Triano had ever seen a subluxation on an x-ray film, he smiled and jokingly replied, "With my eyes closed" [259].

Do Chiropractic Subluxations Cause "Pinched Nerves"?

D.D. Palmer knew that part of B.J.'s "pinched nerve" declaration was palpably false and told him so, to no avail. Even in the earliest part of this century, anatomists knew beyond any shadow of doubt that small misalignments of the vertebrae would not impinge upon spinal nerve roots.

Edmund S. Crelin, Ph.D., a prominent anatomist at Yale University, was deeply offended by the chiropractors' ignorance of human anatomy and incensed by their flamboyant claims. After noting that no one, including chiropractors, had ever experimentally determined how much vertebral displacement is necessary before a spinal nerve is impinged as it leaves the spine, he decided to find out. In the early 1970s, he dissected out the spines, with ligaments attached, from the bodies of six people who had died three to six hours earlier, exposing the spinal nerves as they passed through the openings (intervertebral foramina) between the vertebrae. He wrapped one wire around a spinal nerve, placed another against the inside wall of its passageway, and connected the wires to an ohmmeter so that any contact between the wires would complete a circuit and register on a recorder. After securing each spine in a drill press, he applied measured forces to bend and twist the spine and saw that the nerves were neither impinged (as B.J. Palmer had alleged) nor stretched (as D.D. Palmer had alleged) until the force was

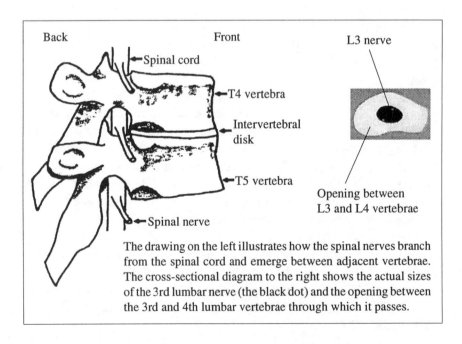

The drawing on the left illustrates how the spinal nerves branch from the spinal cord and emerge between adjacent vertebrae. The cross-sectional diagram to the right shows the actual sizes of the 3rd lumbar nerve (the black dot) and the opening between the 3rd and 4th lumbar vertebrae through which it passes.

great enough to break the spine, an event that would have disastrous consequences in a living person. Crelin reported:

> This experimental study demonstrates conclusively that the sub-luxation of a vertebra as defined by chiropractic—the exertion of pressure on a spinal nerve which by interfering with the planned expression of Innate Intelligence produces pathology—does not occur. [61]

Did this experiment cause chiropractors to discard the Palmers' notions or to sponsor a study of their own to measure how much "misalign-ment" is necessary to cause "nerve impingement"? Hardly. The ACA quickly produced a ten-page document contending that "nerve encroach-ment . . . is a dynamic occurrence and cannot be reproduced in a dead body" [177]. Crelin replied:

> As expected, the president of the American Chiropractic Associa-tion . . . could only conclude that my findings were irrelevant. . . . In one fell swoop he rejected all of the relevant, invaluable medical knowledge acquired from autopsying dead bodies. . . . In a living person there is a reflex response by the powerful spinal muscles to fight or resist any forces that would sublux a vertebra to the degree that it and/or spinal nerves could be damaged. . . . Thus, if the impingement on the nerves could not happen in a dead body, it definitely could not happen in a living one. [60]

Not long afterward, Crelin and several colleagues studied freshly obtained cervical spines and found that the ligaments attached to the cervical vertebrae are very strong and limit their motion and thereby prevent the spinal cord and nerves from being pinched [125].

Of course, spinal nerves *can* be compressed by conditions such as tumors, herniated disks, arthritic joint changes, and bony overgrowths. However, this compression does not cause the body's internal organs to become diseased. If minor pressure occurs, it has little or no effect because nerve impulses are slowed in a zone of partial compression but resume their flow afterward so that the transmitted impulses are normal [24]. When more significant compression occurs, the most common effects are pain, numb-ness, feelings of pins and needles, decreased reflexes, and/or weakness or paralysis of the muscles served by the affected nerves. Moreover, most conditions in which nerves are actually compressed are not appropriate for treatment with manipulation. This has been said for years by medical experts and was recently substantiated by expert panels assembled by the RAND Corporation and the Agency for Health Care Policy and Research (see Chapter 12). RAND's interdisciplinary panel included chiropractors.

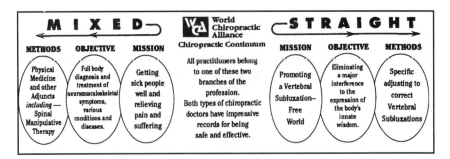

The World Chiropractic Alliance (WCA), a "straight" chiropractic organization, states: "Vertebral subluxation . . . causes alteration of nerve function and interference to the transmission of mental impulses, resulting in a lessening of the body's innate ability to express its maximum health potential." A WCA press kit illustrates this "chiropractic continuum" [44].

What Do Chiropractors Treat?

What chiropractors treat—or say they treat—depends mainly on what they believe. Those who believe that subluxations are the cause of disease, or an underlying cause, tend to claim that the gamut of health problems fall within their scope. Chiropractors who distance themselves from subluxation theory tend to limit their practice to musculoskeletal problems and use manipulation to increase the mobility of joints. As with their theory, some appear to occupy a middle ground.

Chiropractors also vary in how they express their scope. Some display nerve charts suggesting that they can treat the full gamut of disease. Some of these charts (shown in Chapters 2 and 5) relate each level of the spine to a list of diseases and conditions supposedly caused by subluxations at that level. Some chiropractors use less explicit charts showing connections between nerves and body organs. Some use vague wording but attempt to convey the idea that their scope is unlimited. Some use weasel words like "can" and "may" to soften whatever it is that they claim. Others are quite explicit.

Richard E. DeRoeck, D.C., for example, has written a book aptly titled *The Confusion about Chiropractic*, which contains a diagram showing "how a spinal nerve can be pinched by either a disc or vertebra." On the following page he states: "When an organ's nerve supply is compromised over a long enough period of time, disease will develop" [63:67].

A similar viewpoint is expressed in the book *Opportunities in Chiropractic Health Care Careers* (1987), written by R.C. Schafer, D.C., and

Louis Sportelli, D.C., in cooperation with the American Chiropractic Association. (Schafer was a former ACA director of public affairs. Sportelli was an ACA board member who later became board chairman.) Page 49 of the book includes an elaborate illustration from *Gray's Anatomy* that, according to Schafer and Sportelli:

> shows the nerve supply to the vital organs from the brain and spinal cord and suggests the need for maintaining uninterrupted communication through the nerves.
>
> This illustration helps to show that every vital organ is connected with and controlled by nerves from the spinal cord and brain. Through this knowledge, one can more fully understand why chiropractic treatments can relieve so many human ailments.

Inspection of *Gray's Anatomy*, however, does not support this interpretation. The chart merely shows the distribution of *sympathetic* nerves to most of the body's internal organs. *Gray's Anatomy* states that "the sympathetic system generally mobilizes the energy for sudden activity such as that in rage or flight; for example, the pupils dilate, the heart beats faster, [etc.]." Interference with the function of these nerves can influence the various organs in ways that are well known and easy to measure, but this is not related to the development of structural disease. Moreover, there is no evidence that if sympathetic nerves malfunction, chiropractic treatment can normalize their function.

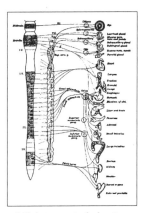

Misinterpreted chart from *Gray's Anatomy*

Sportelli has also written a booklet called *Introduction to Chiropractic: A Natural Method of Health Care*, which has sold millions of copies and is distributed by chiropractors to their patients. The current (ninth) edition states:

> Accidents, falls, uneven stress, tension, over-exertion or any other factor which may cause an inability of the spine to move as a dynamic organ, can result in minor displacements or derangements of one or more of these vertebrae, causing irritation to spinal nerve roots directly by pressure or indirectly through reflexes. These irritations, in turn, may cause malfunctions in your body. Chiropractic teaches that nerve pressure, or nerve reflex can cause a disturbance of delicate body functions resulting in an increased susceptibility to disease processes. [236]

Sportelli contends that "the conditions which doctors of chiropractic treat can be as varied and as vast as the nervous system itself" [236]. But during a recent marketing seminar for chiropractors, he informed the audience:

> I don't happen to think that chiropractic care's for sick people. I think it's for well people to keep 'em well. . . . .We're the only profession that can do something to a patient to ensure wellness before they get sick. . . .
>
> I get adjusted every week, and I have for the last thirty-five years of my life. [237]

The ACA's ad in the March 1988 *Reader's Digest* stated that "functional disorders, such as those that involve organs and glands, may respond to chiropractic adjustments." In April 1994, the ICA placed a full-page ad in the *New York Times* claiming that chiropractic is "a proven alternative to conventional medical care for a wide variety of conditions in children and adults."

Sid Williams, D.C., Life College president and an ICA past-president said in a recent interview, "We do something for everything. . . . Rigor mortis is the only thing that we can't help!" [259]. I don't think he was joking.

"Super-straight" chiropractors—who hold the most explicit Palmerian beliefs—claim that they treat only subluxations, not diseases or even musculoskeletal conditions, and that this enables the body's "Innate Intelligence" to reestablish health. Some maintain this position even though they use the "nerve charts" that cover the gamut of disease. Can you imagine a medical doctor saying, "I only prescribe antibiotics. I don't treat infections"? In 1976, Sherman College of Straight Chiropractic actually published a pamphlet titled "Chiropractors Do Not Treat Disease." A related pamphlet explains:

> The chiropractor does not "fight" the thousands of named diseases. . . . Instead, he or she removes any block to the vital nerve force from the brain through the spinal nerves so that the *Natural Innate Wisdom* (which knows how) may be able to coordinate and balance all the functions of the body. As control is restored, Health . . . will grow and diseases will fade away. [264]

Some chiropractors—mostly the straights—claim that the nervous system is the master of all body functions, regulating everything from major organs to intricate cellular activities. This is absolutely untrue. Although some functions are subject to nervous-system control, others are not. Equally important, the brain and many of the nerves that do affect function are not accessible to spinal manipulation.

A few anatomical facts should help clarify why subluxation theory makes no sense. The only parts of the nervous system conceivably accessible to manipulation are the twenty-six pairs of nerves that exit from the movable segments of the spine. The twelve pairs of cranial nerves that pass through openings in the skull are out of reach, and so are the five pairs that exit through the sacrum, the solid bone formed by fusion of the five vertebrae near the bottom of the spine. The spinal cord is also inaccessible because the vertebrae and other protective tissues surround it.

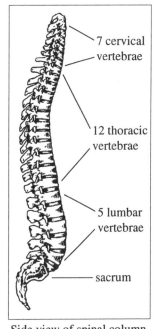

7 cervical vertebrae

12 thoracic vertebrae

5 lumbar vertebrae

sacrum

Side view of spinal column

In addition, many body processes take place automatically. The immune system, for example, is completely independent of the nervous system. In fact, certain immune reactions can take place outside of the body in cell cultures or other laboratory preparations. The heart, stomach, intestines, and blood vessels can be influenced by sympathetic nerves, but their function does not depend entirely upon the nervous system. The stimulus for the heartbeat arises within the heart itself; and the heart, as well as many other organs, can work quite well when transplanted without any direct connection to the recipient's brain, spinal cord, or other nerve tissue. Most biochemical reactions take place automatically at the cellular level and are not influenced by the nervous system. Blood cells have no nerve supply whatsoever.

Additional evidence of independent function comes from observation of individuals who become paraplegic or quadriplegic due to severe injury to their spine. Except for their bladder and large intestine, their internal organs still continue to function. "In short," says Consumers Union, "life can go on despite even massive 'interference' with nerve impulses" [24:171]. Spinal manipulation may stimulate release of endorphins ("natural painkillers") and other hormones that can temporarily influence various body functions, but no such reaction has been proven to prevent or alleviate illness. To responsible physicians—and chiropractors—the aim of manipulation is not to treat disease but to restore normal joint mobility.

Critics of subluxation theory have made some other interesting observations. In 1994, *Consumer Reports* collected information on the practices of more than 250 chiropractors and concluded, "it was clear that the traditional belief system holds sway" [47]. Reformist Samuel Homola, D.C., has noted that "the orthopedic subluxation is an obvious and detectable entity (presenting obvious local symptoms), while the chiropractic subluxation is a theoretical, elusive, and primarily imaginary process to which the chiropractor has attached the primary cause of disease" [107:172]. Reformist Peter Modde, D.C., has pointed out that if chiropractic subluxation theory were correct, people with scoliosis would have every disease mentioned in chiropractic "nerve charts" and quadriplegics could not live. Joseph C. Keating, Jr., Ph.D., an outspoken chiropractic educator, considers the philosophical subluxation a "holy word" that has outlived its usefulness and "will become an increasing embarrassment." But Craig F. Nelson, D.C., another outspoken educator, recently lamented that "the number of chiropractors who are animated by 19th century pseudoscience seems to be growing rather than shrinking, and . . . these chiropractors will abandon their philosophy when hell freezes over" [170]. John Badanes, D.C., a vocal critic of traditional chiropractic, has perhaps the most cutting words:

> Since the beginning. . . chiropractors have tried to sell The Subluxation as The Problem and then sell themselves and their Adjustments as The Solution. The Chiropractic Subluxation is a delusional diagnosis and the Adjustments of Subluxations, by extension, constitute a delusional medicine.
>   The wide spectrum of chiropractic Techniques ALL have their own methods for detecting Spinal Demons and unique methodology for Exorcizing them. Each Technique—AMAZINGLY—will show the potential 'patient' to suffer from Vertebral Subluxation . . . The Silent Killer! [14]

"Innate Intelligence"?

D.D. Palmer introduced his concept of Innate Intelligence (or simply Innate) in an article by that name in 1904. He expanded it in a 1906 book (written with B.J.) and described it fully in his 1910 text [181]. The Palmers maintained that the body's natural healing abilities were linked with a supernatural intelligence. They used this bioreligious concept to explain not only health and disease, but also all of reality. In brief, they contended that "Universal Intelligence" (God) fills the universe and dwells within every living creature in the form of "Innate Intelligence," an organizing force that controls every physical process not under voluntary control [130:28]. This "god within" is the "life force" or "vital energy" that flows from the brain through the spine to every part of the body. Thus the spine (and chiropractors) have great significance because the slightest vertebral misalignment ("subluxation") hinders this divine energy from working freely, which is the true cause of disease. The chiropractor only releases Innate, which actually does the healing.

Joseph H. Donahue, D.C., a student of chiropractic history and philosophy, has criticized this viewpoint as irresponsible:

> The doctor, claiming only to be the "channel" for II [Innate Intelligence], can evade professional accountability. The trick to evading accountability, and yet keeping the patients coming, is to imply a lot of benefits without saying anything specific. Patients never receive an answer to, "Can you help my particular health problem?" "After all," they are told, "chiropractic does not treat disease; it releases the II healing force and the body heals itself." Patients can then be strung along with assurances that the chiropractor is doing everything possible to release the patient's II. There are few outcome measures by which patients can judge their progress. Usual healing arts standards such as symptom relief or improved [laboratory tests] only count partially, if at all. . . . When a patient begins to balk at further care, they can be frightened into continuing care by dire predictions of the "devastating effects of subluxation degeneration." [67]

Besides being spiritual and divine, Innate is also personal, providing supernatural revelations and even making the diagnosis, according to the Palmers and their theosophical disciples. As B.J. put it: "I do nothing. It is Innate that does the work" [13:162]. This "philosophy" was greatly emphasized in the curriculum of the Palmer School of Chiropractic. On page 424 of his book *Answers* (1952), B.J. refers to Innate as the "other fellow," or the "fellow within," and the real originator of chiropractic. In *The Bigness of the Fellow Within* (1949), he stated that "Innate . . . has been building and running millions of bodies for millions of years" and exhorted all chiropractors to harness this divine power. He also said: "One spark of Innate is greater than all the education, books, libraries of man" [178:44]. Today such ideas are maintained most vigorously by "straight" and "super-straight" chiropractors.

Many people caught up in chiropractic think that the theosophical tenets permeating the profession are harmless relics of the past. The truth is, however, that metaphysics still influences chiropractic practice. Donahue laments that the "Innate" concept is still widely taught and perhaps 80 percent of chiropractors still believe in some version of it [67]. Keating is also critical:

These philosophical notions are clearly theological tenets that can only be accepted on faith. As such, they play no role in scientific explanations of chiropractic phenomena, since spirits are outside the realm of the observable and the testable. Concepts like Innate Intelligence, which posits an individual spirit fraction of an infinite God (Universal Intelligence), who guides and directs all functions of the body, do much to retard scientific development. Additionally, chiropractic theological treatises serve to reinforce the cultist, nonscientific image of the chiropractor among other health care professionals and the public. [128]

Sociologist Walter I. Wardwell, Ph.D., describes B.J. Palmer's embrace of Innate as a strategy for survival of the profession [255:183]. Chiropractic's religious tenets made it as different as possible from medicine. This facilitated licensure as a separate health profession and enabled some chiropractors to escape prosecution by claiming they were not practicing medicine. The metaphysical explanation also provided an excuse for not doing research. How can one test for a divine spirit? Of course, the "protection" afforded by Innate has had a negative side as well. Chiropractic is largely marginalized and still shunned by most rational people.

Some people have suggested that "Innate Intelligence" is merely a way to express the concept of homeostasis, the body's ability to protect itself by maintaining its internal balance. However, homeostasis does not involve the flow of supernatural forces or a transfer of energy from one person to another. Nor is there any evidence that misaligned spines interfere with homeostasis or that spinal manipulation enhances it.

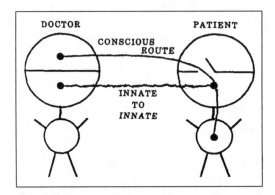

This diagram illustrates what supposedly occurs during Concept Therapy, a widely proselytized chiropractic technique claimed to enable the doctor's Innate Intelligence to communicate with the patient's Innate Intelligence. According to a brochure from the Concept Therapy Institute, "the doctor's thoughts, ideas, and inner feelings are transmitted to the patient vibratorily."

Why Does Subluxation Theory Persist?

I believe that most chiropractors still support chiropractic's original tenets, though many have fudged their language and added other theories in an attempt to justify (or conceal) what they or their colleagues do. In her recent book, *Foundations of Chiropractic: Subluxation*, chiropractic educator Meridel I. Gatterman, D.C., observed:

> The word subluxation has been . . . embodied with a multitude of meanings by chiropractors during the past 100 years. To some it has become a holy word; to others, an albatross to be discarded. . . . To add to the confusion, more than 100 synonyms for subluxation have been used. Why then do we persist in using the term . . . when it has become so overburdened with clinical, political, and philosophical . . . significance . . . that the concept that once helped to hold a young profession together now divides it and keeps it quarreling over basic semantics? The obvious answer is: . . . The concept of subluxation is central to chiropractic. [83:5]

Gatterman is correct that abandoning the "subluxation" would be difficult. There are at least six reasons. First, *subluxation theory and its trappings constitute a delusional system*—a set of false beliefs held despite abundant evidence that contradicts them. Second, the diversity afforded by subluxation theory enables chiropractors to maintain what Dr. William T. Jarvis calls "deniability." No matter what aspect of their behavior is criticized, proponents can always claim that the examples given are not representative of the profession as a whole. Third, if chiropractors disowned their heritage and began thinking and talking the same language as the scientific medical community, chiropractic might not be maintainable as a "separate and distinct" form of practice. Fourth, if chiropractic discarded subluxation terminology, their Medicare coverage might be jeopardized and the state licensing laws that define the practice of chiropractic in terms of "subluxations," "nerve energy," and the like would have to be rewritten. Fifth, if chiropractic schools stopped teaching chiropractic philosophy, their "true believer" alumni might get upset and withdraw financial support. And finally, as discussed in Chapter 17, if the more scientifically oriented chiropractors parted company with the rest, the profession would be weakened politically. As things stand now, chiropractic is clinging for dear life to its cultist and pseudoscientific roots while insisting that it has risen above them.

4

Chiropractic Education
and Licensure

During the past century or so, educational authorities have established an accreditation system whose goal is to foster quality education. At the same time, state governments have passed licensing laws intended to ensure that health-care practitioners are competent.

In the United States, educational standards are set by a network of agencies approved by the U.S. Office of Education (USOE) or the Council on Recognition of Postsecondary Accreditation (CORPA). Almost all of these agencies are voluntary and nongovernmental. Accreditation enables the credits from a school to be transferred to other schools and used as a basis for entering various professions. The Council on Chiropractic Education was recognized as an accrediting agency for chiropractic schools by USOE in 1973 and by CORPA in 1976. Since 1974, when Louisiana passed its chiropractic licensing law, all fifty states have licensed chiropractors. CCE now accredits sixteen of the eighteen chiropractic schools, and almost all state licensing boards require that their applicants be graduates of a CCE-accredited college.

Chapter 2 notes that in 1968 the U.S. Department of Health, Education, and Welfare (HEW) investigated chiropractic teachings and concluded that "the scope and quality of chiropractic education do not prepare the practitioner to make an adequate diagnosis and provide appropriate treatment." This chapter examines the status of chiropractic education today.

What Accreditation Signifies

Academic accreditation constitutes public recognition that an educational program meets the administrative, organizational, and financial criteria of a reviewing body recognized by USOE or CORPA. The accreditation process is intended "to provide a professional judgment as to the quality of the educational institution or program(s) offered, and to encourage the continual improvement thereof" [65]. Accreditation is important not only because it usually signifies high academic standards, but also because it is required for eligibility for federal financial assistance to the school and its students. USOE or CORPA don't accredit individual schools but approve the national and regional agencies that do so.

Recognition of a national or regional agency by the U.S. Office of Education (USOE) is supposed to mean that an agency "is a reliable authority as to the quality of training offered" [65]. The criteria are primarily organizational. To achieve recognition, the agency must be national or regional in its scope and must have appropriate bylaws, procedures, institutional and public representation, "reliability," and autonomy. Individual schools, in turn, must meet criteria set by the recognized agency. However, scientific validity is not among USOE's criteria for approving an accrediting agency for training health-care practitioners! In 1972, when an official from HEW's accreditation staff asked whether the agency's 1968 report on chiropractic was relevant to accreditation, an HEW legal official replied:

> You question whether the Commissioner can judge whether or not to list an accrediting agency for chiropractic education, or any other agency dealing with a field of "questionable legitimacy," on any basis other than its compliance with the criteria published for that purpose.
>
> Under the relevant legislation . . . it is our view that the Commissioner is not called upon to express his opinion as to the legitimacy or social usefulness of the field of training of the agency seeking recognition. That is not to say that where training in the field under question or the practice is patently illegal, or an apparent hoax or fraud, that the Commissioner must recognize . . . an accrediting agency for that subject.
>
> While the Department [HEW] apparently does not feel that the services should be covered under Medicare . . . the training in, or practice of, chiropractic is not outlawed anywhere in the United States. [270]

Under this policy, could chiropractic be disqualified as a fraud or hoax? When an AMA official complained that USOE's policy seemed to be based on the idea that "most states have seen fit to license chiropractic" and that "licensure standards can not redeem chiropractic's scientific invalidity," the U.S. Commissioner of Education replied:

State licensure is relevant . . . *not* because it may (or may not) be tantamount to official recognition of the scientific validity of the field, but *rather* because it seems to take chiropractic out of the exceptional cases—patent illegality, fraud, or hoax—where the Commissioner would be authorized to refuse to recognize . . . an accrediting agency for a discipline. [176]

A few months after this letter was written, Commissioner Terrel H. Bell, Ph.D., granted approval to the Council for Chiropractic Education (CCE). When HEW Secretary Caspar Weinberger concurred, the AMA said Weinberger's decision "threatens to make a mockery of the entire accreditation process" [2]. Indeed it did. Since that time, USOE has recognized accrediting agencies for naturopathy and acupuncture schools that offer an even greater variety of nonsense than is taught at most chiropractic schools. A few years ago, when the naturopathic agency was undergoing evaluation for renewal, a USOE official actually told the National Council Against Health Fraud's attorney Michael Botts that if astrologers could get the required paperwork in order, they could get their own agency for accreditation.

Although independent, CCE was originally formed by the American Chiropractic Association and mainly reflects a "mixer" philosophy. In 1988, USOE approved the Straight Chiropractic Academic Standards Association (SCASA), an accrediting agency formed in 1979 by two "super-straight" (subluxation-based) chiropractic schools. In 1993, however, SCASA's recognition was terminated, leaving CCE clearly in control of chiropractic education. Since graduation from a CCE-accredited school is required for licensure in almost all states, it seems unlikely that any chiropractic college can survive without CCE accreditation.

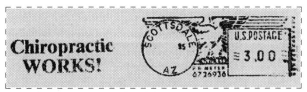

CCE promotes chiropractic with a slogan on its postage meter.

Quantity Does Not Mean Quality

Admission to a CCE-accredited school requires two years of prechiropractic college education with at least a C average. To receive the doctor of chiropractic (D.C.) degree, students must complete a minimum of 4,200 hours of study over a four-year period. The courses include anatomy, biochemistry, microbiology, pathology, physiology, public health, obstetrics, pediatrics, geriatrics, dermatology, otolaryngology, diagnostic imaging procedures, psychology, nutrition/dietetics, biomechanics, orthopedics, first aid and emergency procedures, chiropractic principles and practice, adjustive techniques, research methods, and professional ethics [59]. Chiropractors often suggest that their schooling is similar or equivalent to that of medical doctors, except that chiropractic schools emphasize the management of musculoskeletal disorders rather than treatment with drugs and surgery.

Chiropractic: An Illustrated History notes that "comparisons of course work and required hours were often presented to legislators and public health officials to attest to the quality and intensity of chiropractic education" [190]. Perhaps the most remarkable of these was a tabulation, issued around 1950 by Palmer College, which claimed that its students underwent 4,485 class hours of instruction while medical students at Johns Hopkins had only 3,397. The 3,397 figure translates to about twenty-one hours per week, forty weeks a year, for four years, which seems too low to have been accurate. The Palmer coursework included 195 hours of chiropractic philosophy, sixty-five hours of public speaking, sixty-five hours of training with the neurocalometer and another bogus device, and several other teachings irrelevant to health-care quality. The chart also stated that Palmer students spent more than twice as many hours (520 to 224) learning "diagnosis." Do you think Palmer's students emerged from school with greater diagnostic ability than those from Johns Hopkins?

The most recent "comparison" chart I have seen was published in 1991 by the International Chiropractors Association [265]. It reports 5,222 hours for medical students and 5,112 hours for chiropractic students, but the schools from which these figures were derived are not identified. For public health, the figures are zero hours for medical students and 176 hours for chiropractors—an interesting number considering chiropractic's longstanding *opposition* to public-health measures (see Chapter 14). A more realistic comparison, published in 1990 in the *Journal of Chiropractic Education*, indicates that students at six chiropractic schools averaged 800 total hours in outpatient clinic training, while medical students averaged 2,825 [203].

Most chiropractors claim they can diagnose conditions within their scope and refer the rest to appropriate providers. Is this realistic? Are chiropractors well trained in history-taking, physical examination, and other types of diagnostic testing? Do they have sufficient familiarity with the wide range of human ailments that they can render precise diagnoses? If not, do they have enough experience to be able to tell which symptoms or conditions lie outside their scope? Does the average chiropractor know his or her limitations? Does chiropractic philosophy interfere with the ability to provide appropriate care? Consider the following information.

• Chiropractic students have many hours of classroom training in the basic sciences, but the quality of instruction varies considerably from instructor to instructor and from school to school. Some schools have few instructors with advanced degrees in the subjects that are taught. Even when the basic sciences are taught properly, they have little to do with eventual clinical competence. Anatomy, physiology, biochemistry, and the rest don't prepare students to diagnose and treat patients. They merely prepare students to *study* clinical subjects.

• Clinical training in chiropractic schools is vastly inferior to that in medical schools. Whereas medical school faculties are large and contain experts in virtually every aspect of medical practice, chiropractic schools have little or no input from medical experts.

• Chiropractic students spend far less time than medical students do learning about clinical subjects (the diagnosis and treatment of disease). Whereas medical students see patients encompassing the full range of disease, most patients seen by chiropractic students have musculoskeletal problems. Although some of their courses are based on standard medical textbooks, chiropractic students do not get the clinical experience necessary to make the information meaningful. Chiropractic schooling in such subjects as pediatrics, obstetrics, and gynecology is usually limited to classroom instruction with little or no actual patient contact and no experience with hospitalized patients [168]. One school, for example, has used rubber models to teach students how to perform pelvic and rectal examinations! *The claim that chiropractic school prepares its practitioners to be "primary-care providers" is absurd.*

• CCE requires that students perform a minimum of only twenty-five clinical evaluations. A chiropractic educator has estimated that during their clinical training, chiropractic students typically see only *two* new patients with non-musculoskeletal complaints [168]. Medical students see hundreds of them.

• CCE requires that students interpret a minimum of only twenty-five urinalyses, twenty blood counts (or related procedures), and ten clinical chemistry, microbiology, or immunology tests. Medical students interpret thousands of them.

• Chiropractic textbooks make no effort to debunk the quack practices that are rampant among chiropractic practitioners.

• While most chiropractic students begin practice soon after graduation, the vast majority of medical students pursue three or more years of residency training. This means that physicians starting out usually have two to three times as many years of supervised clinical experience.

• While some students emerge from chiropractic school with a scientific view of health and disease, others do not. Many schools provide what *Consumer Reports* calls "a hefty dose of chiropractic philosophy." Moreover, a significant percentage of students entering chiropractic school have been "raised in chiropractic" and hold rigid misbeliefs about the nature of health, disease, and health care. Although no study has tracked what happens to these beliefs, there is no reason to think they evaporate during chiropractic training.

• Subluxation theory still appears to play a prominent role in chiropractic education. In 1993, *The Chiropractic Journal* sent each of the eighteen chiropractic college presidents a letter containing four questions related to subluxation theory:

1. Does your college teach students to locate and correct vertebral subluxations?
2. Does your college teach students that subluxation correction is the foundation for their practice?
3. Does your college teach students that chiropractic can help conditions other than musculoskeletal?
4. Does your college teach students that subluxations can be identified on x-ray?

Of the fourteen who responded, all but one answered "yes" (or words to that effect) to the first two questions. Most also answered the third question affirmatively, but the presidents of several "straight" schools said their students are taught to treat subluxations rather than diseases or "conditions." Concerning x-ray identification of subluxations, seven said yes and most of the rest said yes, but together with other findings [261]. As far as I can tell, three of the four schools whose presidents declined to answer do not promote subluxation theory to their students.

• Chiropractic students may be exposed to questionable practices through clubs (many schools have "applied kinesiology" clubs, for example) and talks by visiting lecturers. Students are also invited to attend seminars by practice-builders and "technique peddlers." Reformist Michael Dunn, D.C., has reported:

> Within my first few weeks of chiropractic college . . . . I found widespread acceptance among the other students of almost any technique or approach to health care except the use of drugs or surgery. Homeopathy, naturopathy, acupuncture, iridology, colonics, and the central chiropractic "subluxation" premise seemed to be blindly accepted by most students without the least bit of discussion, debate, or call for research evidence. "Medicine" was condemned or disparaged almost daily, not only for organized medicine's alleged "monopolistic" hold on health care, but as a false model and approach to healing! [68]

In a recent commentary, Joseph C. Keating, Ph.D., chiropractic's most persistent academic critic, expressed the problem even more bluntly:

> Several of the largest and some of the smallest student bodies in the profession today are found at institutions that emphasize biotheology, vitalism, pseudo-science, and marketing values. . . . Most in the profession are aware of where the "phooolosophical" leaders in chiropractic education reside. These schools are busy turning out "brand new, old fashioned chiropractors," investigating Innate . . . and "proving" what they always knew was true. . . . And although many graduates of these theological institutions can be expected to reject the most absurd ideas promoted by their presidents and boards, . . . we are faced nonetheless with the alarming reality that a whole new generation of (well meaning) dingbat doctors . . . advertising fanatics, and evangelical ideologists will be with us for many years to come. [129]

Joseph H. Donahue, D.C., has been equally blunt about the teaching of philosophy in chiropractic schools:

> It is all too apparent that many instructors and administrators wouldn't know a "principle" from a prince. That chiropractic colleges continue to graduate too many narrow-minded technicians, avaricious doctors who willingly chant "money, money, money" at seminars, or scientific illiterates is testament to the absence of authentic chiropractic philosophers. That somehow enough individual chiropractors can overcome this educational process and support our creaky scientific superstructure is amazing. [66]

What Licensing Means

It is very common for chiropractors, when questioned as to the legitimacy of what they do, to point out that they are licensed in all fifty states, thus implying that their practices must be scientifically valid. That simply is not true. Licensing is done for purposes of regulation. Licensing laws set minimum requirements for training and knowledge (passage of an exam), but do not specify that practices must be science-based. Even physicians and dentists are not required *by law* to practice according to scientific principles, though they generally choose to do so because their professions are committed to science, which helps to produce quality care. Chiropractic licensing was achieved through political activities in which chiropractors and their patients pressed for legislative endorsement (see Chapter 2).

The percentage of chiropractors practicing in an unscientific and irrational manner is unknown, but is obviously very high. The *majority* of chiropractors responding to the 1991 survey by the National Board of Chiropractic Examiners said they were utilizing one or more of the dubious methods described in Chapters 7 and 8 and the glossary of this book. The percentages reported were: Activator Methods (51.2 percent); applied kinesiology (37.2 percent); nutritional counseling, therapy, or supplements (83.5 percent); acupressure/meridian therapy (65.6 percent); homeopathic remedies (36.9 percent); and acupuncture (11.8 percent) [49]. As far as I know, no chiropractic board has ever disciplined or attempted to stop any chiropractor from doing any of these things. In fact, given these high numbers, it is safe to assume that many board members are using them.

The state laws regulating chiropractic vary considerably. About half are based explicitly on subluxation theory, permitting chiropractors to detect and treat "subluxations" or treat interferences with "nerve energy." Most of the rest permit them to do virtually anything taught in chiropractic schools. Federal laws require that drugs and devices be proven safe and effective before they are marketed or used to treat consumers. No law requires that chiropractic methods meet this standard. Thus, as Consumer's Union has aptly stated, "Current licensing laws . . . lend an aura of legitimacy to unscientific practices and serve to protect the chiropractor rather than the public" [24:183].

The next six chapters describe many of the practices for which public protection is sorely needed.

5

Questionable
Marketing Tactics

It's been said that some people swear by chiropractors and others swear at them. I don't know who authored this insightful comment, but I do understand why it was made. This chapter and the following one examine some of the factors that influence why people develop strong feelings about chiropractors.

Questionable Recruitment Procedures

Many chiropractors use and/or recommend ethically questionable methods for attracting new patients. Peter Fernandez, D.C., former head of a large practice-management firm, has written a series of books called "Secrets of a Practice Building Consultant." The first book in the series, *1,000 & One Ways to Attract New Patients,* contained suggestions like: (a) never go anywhere without being paged; (b) send out thousands of letters to the wrong people, thanking them for referring a patient; (c) hire someone to phone people at random asking for "Dr. So-and-So's office" and plugging his ability to treat headaches; (d) have friends or relatives stop at various places in town asking for directions to your office (to call attention to your name and address); (e) write notes on chiropractic literature with your name on it praising yourself and "lay it all over town"; and (f) pretend you are busier than you are by staging phone calls to your office when patients are there [74].

Many chiropractors advertise that various "danger signals" may indicate a need for chiropractic services. Dr. William T. Jarvis has noted:

> Unlike the American Cancer Society's "Seven Warning Signs of Cancer," which have a scientific basis and are always the same, the lists used by chiropractors have no scientific basis and vary from one practitioner to another. They range from seven to sixteen supposed danger signals and may include more than forty different symptoms, many of which are insignificant and experienced by normal people. Most people who respond to such ads are told that their spine should be adjusted to relieve their symptoms and to prevent future trouble as well. [123]

Free Examinations

Some chiropractors recruit new patients through postural checks and other free screening examinations at health expositions, shopping centers, or other places where there is heavy foot traffic. A large percentage of the people screened are inappropriately advised to have further evaluation or treatment at the chiropractor's office. Dr. Stephen Barrett reported two such experiences in his chapter on chiropractic in *The Health Robbers: A Close Look at Quackery in America:*

> Several years ago, one exhibitor who examined me recommended treatment for excessive tension of my neck (which, if it existed, did not bother me at all). More recently, a chiropractor stated that pains in my left shoulder were caused by a subluxation in my neck and that an immediate $5 deposit would cover the cost of a $75 visit to his office. The actual cause (which I knew) was tendinitis of a biceps muscle that would rub against a shoulder bone when I raised my arm. Soon afterward an orthopedist cured the problem by inserting an instrument into my shoulder and shaving the bone so that the tendon no longer encounters it. [21]

In their offices, some chiropractors perform free initial evaluations that include an x-ray examination, thermography, or contour analysis. Free evaluations are done, of course, with the hope of recruiting long-term patients. Neither thermography nor contour analysis is a valid diagnostic test (see Chapter 7). With respect to the x-ray offer, reformist Samuel Homola, D.C., has cautioned:

> Not everyone needs an x-ray exam. If an individual doesn't have a history of disease or injury and his back pain occurs following a

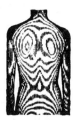
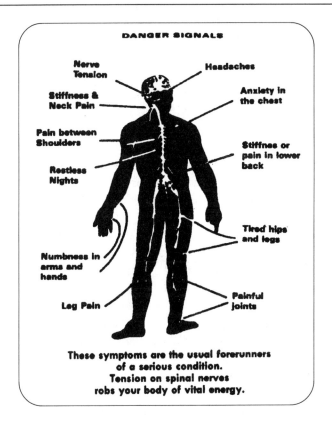
"Danger signal" ads from Yellow Pages. The ads are misleading because: (a) most of the symptoms listed are unlikely to be caused by "pinched nerves," (b) most cases involving the listed symptoms are not serious, and (c) some of the symptoms (such as difficult breathing) are far more likely to be appropriate for *medical* rather than chiropractic evaluation.

simple exertion or after a stumble, chances are it will resolve after a few days or after a few weeks. . . .

Chiropractors who maintain that vertebral misalignment is a cause of disease often x-ray the spine repeatedly in order to adjust specific vertebrae as a preventive measure. . . .

Some of them will x-ray unnecessarily to adjust imaginary or harmless vertebral misalignments, which is a waste of time and money as well as a health risk, especially in the case of infants and children.

The individual who hurts his back and decides to see a chiropractor should not be persuaded into bringing in the whole family for "free exam." And he shouldn't be overly concerned about having misaligned vertebrae that might be surreptitiously damaging to his health. If he does not have pain and he can move around normally, it's doubtful whether he has a vertebra that needs correction by manipulation. [109]

X-ray films are sometimes used to persuade normal people that they have a "spinal curvature" (or not enough curvature, or too much curvature). After "treatment," the curvature "improves" because the patient is positioned differently for the examination.

Many chiropractors have used "nerve charts" relating misalignment or pinching of spinal nerves to diseases of internal organs (see illustrations below and in Chapter 2). The charts contend that spinal manipulation might be helpful for virtually the entire gamut of disease. Explicit claims of that type are no longer common. However, many chiropractors still utilize charts that depict connections between nerves and internal body organs.

Some of these charts are electronic displays that enable chiropractors "at the touch of a button, to colorfully illuminate a subluxated trauma path across its entire spectrum of influence." These products are display boxes whose front panel depicts a cross-section of the body showing the spine and internal organs. Pushing buttons along the spine lights up the supposedly corresponding organs "to create in the patient a higher awareness level of chiropractic benefit." One manufacturer states that "by simply pushing spinal buttons, a patient can create a subluxation and observe . . . . how their subluxations may be connected to organic problems as well as pain."

Such representations are false because "pinched nerves" do not cause organs to become diseased. Moreover, as Homola has noted, impingement is unlikely to occur without obvious signs of trouble:

Spinal nerves are commonly irritated or pinched by herniated discs, bony spurs, and other degenerative changes in the spine. When this happens, there may be pain, numbness, tingling, and other symptoms radiating into musculoskeletal structures supplied by the affected nerves, usually in one arm or leg.

It's thus unlikely to have a pinched nerve without being aware of it. . . .

When a spinal nerve is damaged, weakness and shrinkage may occur in the muscles supplied by the nerve, plus perhaps a loss of sensation and a dysfunction of the circulation in the skin over the muscles. But there is no evidence . . . that the pinching or even cutting of a spinal nerve will affect organic function. Even when the back is broken, the internal organs will continue to function, even though the victim's arms and legs may be paralyzed. . . .

Any time your chiropractor tells you that you have a pinched nerve that might affect your general health, or that you need regular spinal adjustments. . . *don't believe it!* . . .

While spinal manipulation will sometimes relieve the symptoms of a pinched nerve, such treatment might also aggravate a pinched nerve. Any time you have arm or leg pain that is worsened by trial manipulation, discontinue the manipulation and seek the opinion of a neurologist or neurosurgeon. [109]

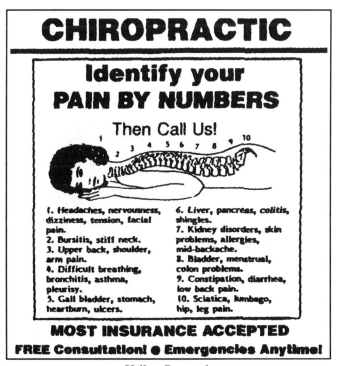

Yellow Pages ad

More Scare Tactics

While doing research for a story on chiropractic, Oliver Fultz was examined by a chiropractor who twice told him, "I know people who've died from subluxations" [81]. The chiropractor called subluxations "silent killers." Then, of course, he advised Fultz to have a course of about fifty spinal adjustments costing $50 each, followed by at least one appointment per month for the rest of his life. A spokesperson for the American Chiropractic Association (ACA) claimed he was "horrified" by Fultz's encounter and contended that it was "anything but typical" and "one of the worst" he had ever seen. But reformist Daniel Futch, D.C., said Fultz's experience was not at all unusual. Warnings against "silent killers" have appeared in many ads, brochures, and office posters, two of which are pictured below. And recommendations for lifetime "maintenance care" are not rare.

Several years ago, the Vertebral Subluxation Research Institute (VSRI) was launched by Terence Rondberg, D.C., of Chandler, Arizona, who is also president of the World Chiropractic Alliance and publishes a newspaper called *The Chiropractic Journal.* VSRI taught how to recruit volunteers for "research" and convert them into patients. To attract chiropractors to its program, it ran ads asking, "Can you fit 20 new patients into your schedule this month?" Respondents received a videotape in which clients told how much the program had built their practice and how they had recovered their initial investment within a few weeks. The program was based mainly on

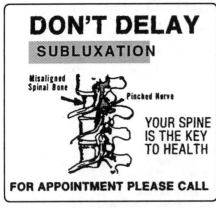

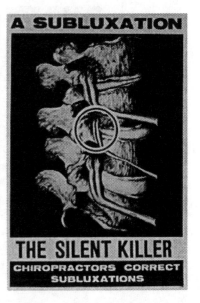

The ad above is from a recent Yellow Pages. The picture on the right is a poster currently sold by a company that calls it "the most powerful single visual aid available."

telemarketing to recruit "research volunteers," who would be converted, if possible, into "lifetime patients"—even if they had no symptoms. Some of the solicitations were directed to people involved in auto accidents whose names were obtained from police reports.

During the first visit, patients completed a questionnaire that included sketchy questions about emotional status, diet, exercise activities, alcohol and tobacco habits, health history, family data, and income. (The questions covered only a tiny portion of what a competent physician would ask in a medical or lifestyle history.) Next, patients were asked to read a brochure explaining the supposed dangers of subluxations ("The Silent Killer") and the chiropractor's role in correcting them. Then came a spinal examination, followed—in most cases—by an x-ray exam. The second visit was a "report of findings" to discuss the "subluxations or other spinal conditions for which chiropractic would be beneficial." Noting that people without symptoms often show "definite evidence" of subluxations, the manual suggested telling them that chiropractic treatment might prevent future trouble.

VSRI claimed that the purpose of its program was to explore possible connections between "subluxations" and various lifestyle factors. Even if that were true, the data generated by such a study would be meaningless because the participating chiropractors diagnosed "subluxations" in different ways. After both the American Chiropractic Association and the International Chiropractors Association denounced "patient research/solicitation schemes," VSRI disappeared from view.

Care to Have a Checkup?

How often should people who feel well have their spine examined and adjusted? In 1979, representatives of the Lehigh Valley Committee Against Health Fraud (LVCAHF) posed that question to thirty-five local chiropractors in Allentown, Pennsylvania, and nearby communities. Almost all recommended at least one checkup per year. The majority gave answers in the range of four to twelve times a year.

The American Chiropractic Association says that one of the best ways to guard your health is through periodic spinal examinations: "Check your calendar and see how long it has been since you and every member of your family had a spinal examination. If several months have elapsed . . . make an appointment." A recent pamphlet warns that "the result of an innocent twist, turn, lift or awkward postural position may cause a spinal subluxation which, if not corrected, can interfere with functions of your nervous system and result in serious illness" [9]. Another pamphlet advises: "Vacations are conducive to situations that may cause spinal misalignment. . . . It is wise to have a chiropractic spinal examination before you leave and after you return" [246].

Another tactic used to motivate patient compliance is to warn of irreversible damage if a long course of manipulative treatment is not begun immediately. The experience of Harriet Cressman, detailed by Dr. Barrett, is a shocking example [21]. After seeing a chiropractor regularly for ten years for "preventive maintenance," she was suddenly informed that her x-ray showed "eighteen compressed discs and progressive osteoarthritis of the spine that was spreading rapidly." She paid $10,000 up front for five months of "intensive" treatment that the chiropractor said was necessary to avoid becoming a helpless cripple. The chiropractor also persuaded Harriet to bring her son in for an exam. He was told that he had a "pin dot of arthritis which, if untreated, would spread like wildfire and leave him crippled within a short time." When the chiropractor suddenly dumped them with the intention of leaving the state, the Cressmans consulted the county district attorney, who advised them to file charges of theft by deception. The D.A.'s office found that several other patients had undergone similar experiences, and a medical radiologist who x-rayed the spines of Harriet and her son offered to testify at trial that neither had any condition that could possibly be helped by chiropractic treatment. Rather than face prosecution, the chiropractor returned the Cressmans' money.

Dire warnings are also being directed to parents about the health of their children. The three-hundred-page *Chiropractic Pediatric & Prenatal Reference Manual*, published by a chiropractic supply house called The Baby Adjusters, advises chiropractors that, "*Now* is the time to tell your patients that subluxations are slowly killing their children. The time is *now* to start adjusting children from birth." The book also says, "Every time a child receives a chiropractic adjustment it should be given as if their very life depends on it, because it does." The foreword states:

> Thousands of infants and children die every week because they never receive chiropractic care. Who is at fault? Is there any parent, who if they truly understood the [chiropractic] principle, would not knock down your door to have their dying baby checked for subluxations? [187]

Practice-Building

Chiropractic is notorious for its patronage or tolerance of deceitful marketing tactics taught by practice-building firms whose primary purpose is to vastly increase the volume of patients, often regardless of any objective need for treatment. Some marketing firms do engage in legitimate office-management analysis and streamlining, but others teach questionable marketing techniques that have little to do with the quality of treatment and a whole lot to do with making more money. Reformist Mark Sanders, D.C., has noted:

> Some advise their clients that "every patient needs a minimum of 30 visits" and they also recommend a certain number of x-rays per patient.
> Leaf through a few chiropractic publications, and you'll find practice-builders hawking "detailed steps for the $40,000-per-month practice," and plans for boosting patient volume by 450 visits a month, or to more than 350 a day. Hundreds of practitioners subscribe to such programs. To help them sustain the money-making momentum, some practice-building firms actually hold meetings to give their clients awards based on increased practice profits. [209]

Dr. William Jarvis describes chiropractic "practice-builders" as "success promoters who train chiropractors in psychological patient manipulation" [120]. Even sociologist Walter I. Wardwell, a staunch chiropractic supporter, has commented on "practice-building entrepreneurs whose programs attract too much attention and are often transparent gimmicks for exploiting patients" [256:186]. Wardwell's treatise on chiropractic history notes that "one motivating technique reportedly used at a school and in seminars is to have all the participants simultaneously hum: 'M-M-M-M' (for 'money')!" [255:271]. I consider this practice a formalized promotion of greed.

Ten years ago, the Parker Chiropractic Research Foundation (PCRF), the largest of the practice-builders, boasted that over two-thirds of all practicing chiropractors had attended its seminars, resulting in "at least a billion dollars of extra chiropractic earnings!" [216]. Its founder, James W. Parker, D.C., advises chiropractors to "Lather Love Lavishly" (to do many things to make patients feel that you really care about them).

Share International, PCRF's chiropractic supply house, sells a huge line of equipment, forms, books, recordings, pamphlets, inspirational literature, charts, greeting cards, plaques, and other practice-management and practice-building aids. Among them are several "report of findings" forms on which the chiropractor can indicate the subluxated areas and the number of recommended visits. One such form is pictured below.

During the late 1960s, Parker and Share International achieved

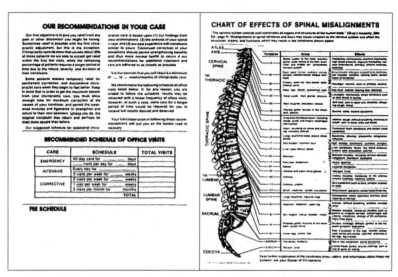

Inside pages of a four-page Share International form—sold during the 1980s—for presenting the chiropractor's findings and recommendations to the patient. The chart falsely claims that "spinal misalignments" can cause crossed eyes, abscessed tonsils, pneumonia, jaundice, and many other health problems. The currently sold version of this form names few diseases but uses physiological-sounding gobbledegook to suggest that nerve-root irritation and compression are somehow related to many symptoms, including "various and numerous symptoms from trouble or malfunctioning" of the heart, thyroid, liver, and a dozen other organs.

considerable notoriety after investigative reporter Ralph Lee Smith attended a Parker seminar and exposed what he observed. One technique taught at the course was to offer a free consultation but, during the same visit, to lead patients into an examination that costs money. Seminar attendees were taught about the "Yet Disease" and "digging for chronicity." As described in Smith's book *At Your Own Risk*:

> "If the patient has a pain in his left shoulder," Dr. Parker said, "ask, 'Has the pain started in your right shoulder yet?' Use it when you must instill a sufficient amount of fear to get the patient to take chiropractic."
>
> The next step is to "dig for chronicity." The doctor puts an elaborate series of questions to the patient that suggest or imply that the condition is chronic. [232:43]

Parker's 336-page *Textbook of Office Procedure and Practice Building for the Chiropractic Profession* states that the "minimum time for maximum possible correction [of spinal misalignments] is an average of one adjustment for each millimeter of misalignment." The book suggests that chiropractors base their treatment recommendation on this "semi-scientific calculation" as well as the patient's history, time for educating the patient, "your judgment," "healing time for organs and tissues involved," "healing time for injured or irritated nerves involved," and the fact that "one adjustment for each year of age of the average chronic patient over 20 years of age is a rough thumbnail guide of what people will willingly accept and pay for" [184:147]. Promoting rehearsed salesmanship, the book lists eighty-four "sentences that sell chiropractic and you" and ninety-four advertising phrases that are "clearly explanatory, persuasive, convincing, and will prompt action!" These include:

- Regular chiropractic care maintains your resistance to disease at the highest possible level.

- The best health insurance you'll ever buy is regular adjustments of your spine, releasing nerve pressures.

- Chiropractic is not limited . . . as a health service to any few particular diseases, because it searches for and removes causes, rather than treats effects.

- Chiropractic searches for, and removes, causes of diseases . . . rather than treats effects. That is why chiropractic has been success-ful, many times after all other methods of healing have failed.

- When the CAUSE of disease or pain has been removed, normal or natural health is the inevitable result.

Many chiropractors utilize materials that reinforce the idea of a special bond between themselves and their patients. The bumper sticker below was distributed by the American Chiropractic Association. The heart sticker is from a company that sells novelty items to chiropractors. Several companies sell birthday cards and other greeting cards with chiropractic themes.

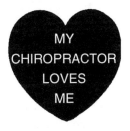

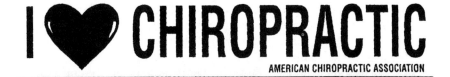

• It is not true to say that you have done everything possible unless modern, scientific chiropractic was included.

• If given half a chance, NATURE will heal and mend any sick body.

The book also advises chiropractors to divert patients "from the muddy road of medicine to the superhighway of chiropractic."

Sid E. Williams, D.C., another chiropractic college president who has run practice-building seminars, has also recommended the "Yet Disease" ploy. His book, *Dynamic Essentials of the Chiropractic Principle, Practice and Procedure*, advises chiropractors to feel the spine for tender spots, "predict the conditions that might occur underneath," and ask whether various symptoms have yet occurred, and if the patient answers no to any of these symptoms, to say:

> Well, Mrs. Jones, it certainly is a wonder. I must say you have a strong constitution in order to stand up under the many problems that you have. You have trouble in many areas, but you don't have many symptoms as of yet. But I would make the prediction that if you hadn't turned to chiropractic, you'd be a very sick girl shortly. [267:98]

The book notes that telling patients they look better may inspire them to tell their friends that chiropractic is helpful. But it advises chiropractors to be careful which words they use:

> Keep in mind that we don't want to feature "Well" or "Cure" too soon or too strongly because the patient won't show up for the next visit since he thinks "I'm ready to quit; I am well." He is never well—just better. Don't emphasize improvement too fast. Instead we say, "We want to get you over on the good side of the ledger and keep you there." [267:216]

F. Michael Anderson, D.C., a practice-builder said to have billed over $40,000 monthly in the mid-1980s, has advised chiropractors to include a long-range treatment plan in their report of findings. In a book described as "the first complete practice building manual to be written by chiropractors for chiropractors," he stated:

> The doctor who does not offer planned care is, basically, treating symptoms. These patients can be expected to be discharged after 1–10 visits. If the patient has any degree of spinal degeneration, this rationale will be inadequate for total health welfare. Also, this doctor must see a high volume of new patients just to survive.
>   On the other hand, patients who clearly understand the concept of spinal degeneration and subluxation complex are those most

likely to refer others to their caring doctor and to follow through with enthusiasm their assigned schedule of treatment. This produces a more stable and stronger practice, and accounts for ultimate success. [5]

The ACA has said that the key to practice growth is to turn satisfied patients into enthusiastic patients who refer. Its 1984 practice-development textbook states that the development of a referral practice is not just the application of techniques but the result of an office's philosophy. "As such," the manual notes, "the philosophy enters into and colors all financial, administrative, technical, clinical, and human relations functions of the practice" [213:284]. Its recommendations include: (1) impress your patients with the results they have realized; (2) suggest chiropractic health care when anyone mentions a sick or disabled friend or relative; (3) have a system of motivational communications, such as thank-you cards and congratulatory notes; (4) "when patients are at their peak of enthusiasm," suggest that they mention chiropractic to their friends, relatives, neighbors, and associates; and (5) patronize worthy patients who are attorneys, dentists, optometrists, druggists, retailers, insurance agents, contractors, etc., even if you can obtain the same services slightly cheaper at another location. In other words, wherever you go, sell yourself and suggest that you might be able to help everyone.

Brainwashing?

Another practice-builder who has developed an elaborate set of sales techniques is David Singer, D.C., whose activities are described in Chapter 6. In an article titled "Effective Patient Retention," he states:

No average person is going to drop his medical belief system in a ten-minute discussion. The only way you get someone to understand chiropractic is to spend time, visit after visit, explaining the basic concept: The body can heal itself when free from nerve interference. [231]

The following accounts illustrate the potency of chiropractic indoctrination.

• A married couple and their twenty-four-year-old daughter were going to the same chiropractor back in the late 1950s. During one of the mother's sessions of neck manipulation, she experienced sudden paralysis of both arms, as well as some other symptoms of a vertebrobasilar stroke. Undaunted, the daughter went to the chiropractor just three weeks later and

Portion of a recent newspaper ad by a Pennsylvania chiropractor. The ad offered an initial examination "including x-ray and consultation if necessary . . . (a $150.00 value)" for $29.00.

during neck manipulation suffered complete paralysis of one arm, dizziness, vomiting, slurred speech, and visual disturbances indicative of a stroke. Incredibly, two months after the daughter recovered, the father also suffered a stroke at the chiropractor's hands [34].

• Early in 1994, ABC's "20/20" aired a thirty-minute segment on chiropractic pediatrics in which they described a married couple whose child became paralyzed hours after spinal manipulation by their chiropractor. They actually took their paralyzed boy back to the chiropractor believing that more manipulation might relieve the paralysis.

Violations of Trust

It is little wonder that the U.S. Inspector General's 1986 report on chiropractic referred to "patterns of activity and practice which at best appear as overly aggressive marketing—and, in some cases seem deliberately aimed at misleading patients and the public regarding chiropractic care" [167]. The cheap hucksterism reminiscent of B. J. Palmer is deeply embarrassing to chiropractors who are interested in the scientifically appropriate use of spinal manipulation and whose highest priority is quality patient care. Reformists like Charles E. DuVall, Jr., D.C., and Daniel Futch, D.C., believe that the sleazy marketing tactics described in this chapter are forms of ritualized patient abuse motivated mainly by greed. If the chiropractors who use them believe their services are valuable, why must they resort to trickery?

6

"Preventive Maintenance"

Many chiropractors contend that everyone needs regular spinal adjustments to optimize nerve function and thereby prevent disease. Chiropractors refer to this process as "preventive maintenance" (or "preventative maintenance"). The idea behind it is that periodic examinations of the spine can detect "subluxations" in their early stages, enabling the chiropractor to correct them. The basic sales pitch is a "carrot-and-stick" approach, predicting benefit for patients who have preventive-maintenance adjustments and trouble for those who don't.

Persuasive Techniques

How can patients be persuaded to come once a month (or once a week) for life? The most complete treatise on this subject is probably *Dynamic Essentials of the Chiropractic Principle, Practice and Procedure*, a 254-page manual distributed during the 1970s [267]. Its author, Sid E. Williams, D.C., is president of Life College (the largest chiropractic school) and a former president of the International Chiropractors Association (ICA). Williams appears to believe that virtually all health problems are caused by nerve interference treatable by chiropractic methods. The manual contains detailed instructions on how to persuade patients to undergo lifetime care. It divides the initial phase of patient contact into three parts: the consultation, the examination (including an x-ray exam of every patient), and the report of findings. Page 129 states:

Every step of your procedure should be thorough enough to convince the patient that you are not overlooking anything. The sophisticated age in which we live prevents the simplicity of chiropractic from being understood by the average person. . . .

The examination procedures are not diagnostic, they are to emphasize to the patient that a weakness exists in his body and that they have been caused by spinal fixations. By fortifying the patient's knowledge of the 'spinal cause' by the use of test instruments and graphs, the patient is able to see beyond any doubt that he is actually physically sick, that a spinal condition caused it, and that something needs to be done chiropractically to correct it.

Williams recommends that after the initial symptoms are relieved, the patient should be persuaded to continue "preventive maintenance" on a monthly basis. (Page 75 notes that "once the patient has experienced relief through chiropractic adjustments, he will accept almost any reasonable recommendation.") If the patient asks, "But will I have to continue with chiropractic care as long as I live?" the recommended reply (page 175) is:

(Chuckling) No ma'am, you won't have to continue it as long as you live. Only as long as you want to stay healthy. Every spine needs some maintenance, Mrs. Jones. My family and I are checked regularly on a monthly basis, and more often when we think that it is necessary. Yes, if you want to stay healthy, you will have to continue some chiropractic care.

In 1979, Williams appeared on CBS's "60 Minutes," adjusting the neck of an infant girl. When asked why, her mother said the adjustments (begun on the child's third day of life) were "preventative measures—to keep her healthy."

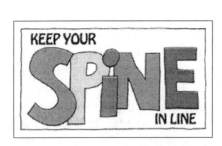 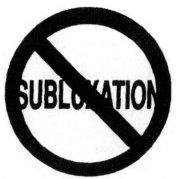

Many office supply companies sell novelty items designed to reinforce the chiropractic message. The item on the left is used for appointment and business cards. The one on the right is a sticker.

The *ICA Practice Management Manual* states that the goal of the second visit (report of findings) is to convert the new patient into a "chiropractic patient." It explains:

> The chiropractic patient is a layman who has come to you with a health problem and has changed his opinion about health and disease and what to do about them. In all probability this person was medically oriented. Since birth he has likely been exposed to medical propaganda, which convinced him that whenever he has had a pain, symptom, or disease the first thing he wanted is relief. Once relief has been found through medication, the care is completed.
>
> After the patient's acceptance of chiropractic, this individual thinks of chiropractic as a valuable aspect of health care. The patient knows that if he is unhealthy, he/she must undergo chiropractic care to normalize the body and free it of nerve impulse interference so that it can function normally. [185]

Frank J. King, Jr., N.D., D.C., a homeopathic manufacturer whose products are discussed in Chapter 7, has likened the initial patient contacts to a love affair:

> The history and consultation period is like a courtship. This is the time when your patients develop, in the back of their minds, the depth of commitment to you, the doctor.
>
> The examination can be compared to the engagement, and the report of findings to the wedding or final ceremonial. If the correct emphasis is placed on a thorough history and the appropriate examination and lab tests, then the report of findings simply falls into place like a smooth wedding ceremony. All the tension of the doctor and the patient is eliminated, and there is no need to attempt a "sales job" on the patient. [135]

In a recent article, Michael Schneider, D.C., severely criticized chiropractors for making unsubstantiated claims for "preventive maintenance." But he also stated that the concept might not be completely wrong:

> Many maintenance patients are not coming regularly because they think they can prevent spinal decay, but for a much simpler reason: It feels good. Patients frequently report that they feel less muscle tension and an enhanced sense of well-being after a chiropractic visit, and that has value in today's fast-paced, stress-filled world. [215]

Singer Enterprises, a practice-management firm in Clearwater, Florida, offers a large line of subluxation-based instructional materials for

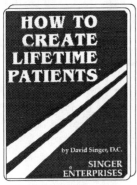

Audiotape set from
Singer Enterprises

chiropractors, their staff, and their patients. Company president David Singer, D.C., teaches that chiropractors will render greater service and achieve a "more successful, low-stress practice" if they become adept at retaining patients when their insurance runs out or their symptoms are gone [231]. His audiotape set called "How to Create Lifetime Patients" advises chiropractors not to tell patients the results of their initial exam or how long they'll need treatment until they've been indoctrinated into the benefits of lifelong chiropractic care. According to a recent company newsletter:

Patient retention comes as a result of education. . . . There is usually only one reason why your patients don't continue to receive the chiropractic care they need: They don't understand what a subluxation is and its effects. . . .

We must educate patients so that they understand that chiropractic care is a part of life; once subluxations are corrected, the body will innately heal itself. [153]

Singer teaches that "only the consumer who understands nerve interference will pay cash after his symptoms are gone" [231]. How should this "understanding" be accomplished? He recommends offering "relief care," "corrective care," and "maintenance care." His "Relief Care" pamphlet states:

Relief care is that care necessary to get rid of your symptoms . . . but not the cause of it. It is the same as drying a floor that was getting wet from a leak, but not fixing the leak.

Corrective care differs . . . in that its goal is to get rid of the symptoms . . . while correcting the cause of the problem as well.

Singer advises that when "correction" has been achieved, patients should be encouraged to pay an annual fee for maintenance care, with visits as often as needed. His "Maintenance Care" pamphlet explains:

Q. Why does a person need Health Maintenance?
A. Maintenance care is made necessary by the stresses of living.
Q. How does Health Maintenance work?
A. It works to remove the cause of problems before symptoms arise or serious conditions show themselves.
Q. What are the benefits?

A. You feel better, increase endurance and reduce the risk of health problems.

Q. When should you start?

A. As soon as corrective care is complete.

Q. Who needs Health Maintenance?

A. Anyone who wants the most out of life.

Singer further advises that it is a mistake to sell patients a three-month course of treatments; "lifetime" care is the goal, so you have to regularly explain that "nerve interference will remain and people need adjustments because nothing else really works to make people well."

In a practice-building manual published in 1985, Micheil W. Hanczaryk, D.C., wrote that "the person who exhibits no symptoms is not necessarily healthy, but rather . . . could be dying a slow death because of their vital force being cut off or altered." He advised chiropractors:

A measure of a successful chiropractic practice is the number of patients returning on a once-a-month, twice-a-month basis, or whatever you consider to be maintenance. These are the people that really know what chiropractic is all about. . . .

You simply must stop practicing relief care. That's not chiropractic, that's medicine. It's far better that people see a medical doctor if they only want Rolaids (or relief). But if it's a cure they want, you are the person for them.

How do we turn that around?

First, do not set up a treatment plan revolving around pain.

Next, get patients committed to a next appointment time. Either the next day, week, month, or whatever they need. . . . The only active patients you have are the ones with an appointment in the book. If you allow a patient to leave the clinic without an appointment, you are cheating them and killing them. [99]

R.C. Herfert, D.C., has written a booklet about the "vertebral subluxation complex" ("VSC") to help chiropractors collect their fees from insurance companies. The booklet states:

Periodic examinations and proper care in the initial stages of disease prevent the development of a serious and extensive problem. . . .

Preventive and/or maintenance care consists of periodic screenings of non-clinical patients who have shown a previous VSC or a predisposition to a VSC. . . . It is also performed as a public service for civic groups, school children and the general public during spinal health care days at schools, shopping centers and malls.

SUBLUXATION PATTERNS
BIOMECHANICAL SUBLUXATION COMPONENT

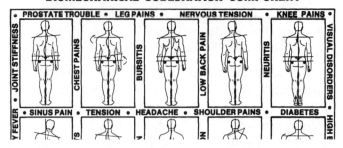

Portion of a chart relating twenty "subluxation patterns" to chest pains, deafness, depression, epilepsy, flu, heart trouble, liver disorders, visual disorders, and forty other diseases and conditions. The chart, which contains no directions for use, occupies a full page in the booklet "Communicating the Vertebral Subluxation Complex," published in 1986 by Herfert Chiropractic Clinics.

Several years ago, a flyer for Herfert's "continuing education seminars" said he had been in practice for more than twenty-five years and had personally given more than one million adjustments. (To generate such a number working six days a week, he would have had to do about 120 adjustments per day.) The illustration above is part of a chart in his booklet.

Back Talk Systems, of Colorado Springs, Colorado, specializes in "chiropractic communication tools that fit into just about any practice, regardless of technique, philosophy, or procedure." Its 1995 catalog advises that "if only a fraction of all the patients you'd ever seen, were still showing up once or twice a month (or as often as *you* get checked), your new patient problems would be over." Its "Welcome to Chiropractic" video advises patients to "think of chiropractic as orthodontics for the spine." Its "Report of Findings" video advises that "abnormal motion or position of spinal bones is like a car that needs a front-end alignment." Its "Chiropractic Lifestyle" video states that "spinal degeneration can be preventable" and features "inspirational testimonials" from actual patients who explain why they've continued regular maintenance care. Back Talk's "Subluxation Degeneration" poster contains a series of x-ray films and suggests that regular spinal checkups can prevent "spinal decay" if care is begun while the spine is "textbook normal."

Back Talk's "Continue Care Postcards" contain brief messages to send patients during the early stages of their care. One, which pictures a sailboat, urges the patient to stay on course. Another, which depicts a pothole, states that patching ("again and again") rarely fixes the underlying

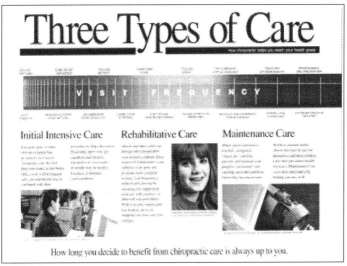

Poster from Back Talk Systems

problem. Another likens investing in chiropractic care to a program of consistent "piggy bank" savings. The fourth states that crooked teeth will resume their crooked position if braces are removed too soon, and "Same with your spine!" if chiropractic treatment is stopped too soon. The company also offers a "Three Types of Care" poster (promised to reduce patient dropout), and referral posters (to encourage patients to refer others).

Consumer Reports describes preventive maintenance as "a hallowed chiropractic tradition" [47]. Many chiropractors who recommend it have their own spine checked and "adjusted" regularly by a colleague. In some cases, their beliefs were solidified before they became chiropractors. During a recent visit to Los Angeles Chiropractic College (which does *not* espouse "subluxation" theory), Dr. Stephen Barrett had an opportunity to chat with a group of twenty students. Four said they had their spine adjusted once a month, and four said they had it done weekly!

The American Chiropractic Association says that one of the best ways to guard your health is through periodic spinal examinations. "Check your calendar and see how long it has been since you and every member of your family had a spinal examination. If several months have elapsed . . . make an appointment." The International Chiropractors Association says: "Even if you feel fine, chiropractic care can help your body maintain its required level of health and fitness. . . . Regular spinal checkups can help detect spinal stress due to subluxations" [72]. Neither group appears to have a current policy statement on the issue of monthly or weekly visits for "preventive maintenance."

Critical Comments

Can periodic detection and correction of "subluxations" do anything for people's health? There is certainly no scientific support for this belief, and most people's experience argues strongly against it, since those without regular chiropractic treatment do quite well for long periods of time. The bulk of twentieth-century medical knowledge testifies against chiropractic's tenaciously held dogma and the basic subluxation theory upon which the concept of preventive maintenance rests. It also stands to reason that if preventive maintenance were cost-effective, insurance companies would encourage it to boost their profits. As far as I know, they all reject the idea.

Has anyone actually tested whether "preventive maintenance" improves general health or prolongs life? As far as I know, no scientific comparison has been made between people who undergo it and people who don't.

Some enlightened chiropractors have made critical observations. Mark Sanders, D.C., who practiced privately for a decade and taught at a chiropractic college for three years, states, "I'm not aware of any scientific proof that spinal manipulations have a preventive effect, yet I've reviewed hundreds of cases in which patients received them without documented complaints of pain or significant objective findings" [209]. He says this is treatment of "nonexistent problems." Scott Haldeman, D.C., M.D., Ph.D., a neurologist who is also a third-generation chiropractor, affirms that "there are no long-term outcome trials on the value of preventive chiropractic care" [47].

Preventive manipulation is scientifically legitimate when used to anticipate patterns of muscle tension and spasm caused by certain types of trauma that can result in immobility of the spine. For example, head injury (including concussion) can result in restriction of movement in the neck. Neurologist Karel Lewit found that fifty-nine of sixty-five of his patients with concussion had clinical abnormalities in the cervical spine, usually between the top two segments [145:350]. Of course, his cervical manipulations do not involve the dangerous thrusting techniques used by some chiropractors. In most cases, gentler (mobilization) techniques are effective and one treatment is sufficient. According to Lewit, certain internal diseases can cause restrictions in spinal mobility that can be anticipated and treated in their earliest stages. He states loss of neck mobility can result from awkward positioning of the head during general anesthesia [145:351].

Such prudent and judicious use of manipulation for preventive purposes is worlds away from what goes on in chiropractic offices where symptom-free patients are indoctrinated to come monthly or weekly throughout their lifetime. Consumers Union has described unwarranted "preventive" care as a way to "fleece healthy people as well as sick people" [24:17]. Many years ago, reformist Samuel Homola, D.C., pointed out that patients can be made overdependent:

> There is considerable difference between the symptoms of . . . patients manipulated by the chiropractor for "the removal of nerve interference" and the symptoms of an acutely locked vertebral joint. The majority of the "subluxations" commonly found by many chiropractors are likely to be painless and imaginary. In replacing these imaginary subluxations, the practitioner places his hands on the patient's back and applies a sudden thrust. . . . This thrust, with "popping" of the vertebrae, has a tremendous psychological influence over the mind of the healthy patient as well as over the mind of the sick patient. . . . [Popping, like "cracking" of the knuckles, simply reflects a sudden separation of joint surfaces held in close contact by fluidic attraction in a vacuum; it has nothing to do with a bone being "put back in place."] . . . Such treatment used on the mentally unstable and nervous person can cause a great deal of harm . . . by perpetuating a psychosomatic condition or even creating a new psychological illness. . . .
>
> Under the typical chiropractic examination, there is no one, at any time, who will not present "one or more subluxated vertebrae" in his spine. Thus, a chiropractic patient often becomes a lifetime patient.
>
> Needless to say, the vertebrae will continue to "pop" as long as an effort is made to do so, which, in the patient's mind, indicates that a person is never quite safe from the ravages of disease unless he continues to take regular chiropractic adjustments. For this reason, many healthy people submit excessively to spinal manipulation in order to "stay healthy." [107:95]

Similar observations have been made by Ralph C. Cinque, D.C., of Buda, Texas, who considers himself a "chiropractic heretic":

> There is no more benefit to back cracking than there is to knuckle cracking, but, unfortunately, the potential for harm is much greater. . . . The spine is strong, but it is also a delicate neuro-muscular mechanism. Applying force to it is like trying to adjust a wristwatch with a sledgehammer.
>
> You will observe that people who get adjustments are the ones who always seem to need them. They are the ones who often feel like "something is out" in their neck or back. Such an idea never occurred to them before they started getting adjustments. Most

people go through their whole life without ever thinking such a thing, or experiencing such an urge. But once the idea is instilled in them by a chiropractor, that they need the adjustments, it can be very difficult for them to shake the obsession. People become *addicted* to chiropractic adjustments, and that is reason enough to avoid them. When a chiropractor isn't handy, they start popping their own necks—a most disturbing sight indeed. [52]

In a recent article in *Dynamic Chiropractic*, Michael Schneider, D.C., warned his colleagues that "preventive maintenance" claims can make the entire profession look bad:

Where is the proof that chiropractic care can prevent or reverse spinal degeneration? We have no hard data to back up this claim and put ourselves in a precarious position by blatantly stating that we can prevent degenerative joint disease. One day soon, with all the media attention we have been receiving, some smart reporter or research "expert" is going to ask for substantiation of these claims. We are going to be publicly embarrassed when cases of patients who were under monthly chiropractic care were actually made worse while undergoing treatment. . . .

We need to recognize that chiropractic treatment for patients who are asymptomatic is risky business, because if they do develop a problem during the course of maintenance care . . . patients may lose confidence in the chiropractic profession. [215]

Andrew Weil, M.D., a staunch proponent of "alternative" health care, has also expressed concern:

Chiropractors are quite successful in making patients dependent on them. I have never heard of a patient being told he or she has a normal spine on a first visit to one of these practitioners. There are always subluxations. Most patients are told they must come in for regular manipulation to make the adjustment "hold." The tendency of chiropractors to seduce patients into long and costly therapy without promoting self-reliance smacks of the style of B.J. Palmer, who even came up with a formula for determining the number of visits to try for based on a patient's age and annual income. [258:132]

The bottom line is that periodically manipulating the spine of healthy people has no proven benefit and involves some risks of physical and psychological injury as well as financial injury.

7

Dubious Diagnostics
and Therapeutics

The American Chiropractic Association would like you to believe that chiropractors adhere to the same diagnostic and treatment standards as medical doctors. According to its booklet *Chiropractic: State of the Art:*

> The doctor of chiropractic conducts a systematic and thorough physical examination using the methods, techniques, and instruments that are standard with all health professions. In addition, a postural and spinal analysis is included.
>
> The chiropractor uses the standard procedures and instruments of physical and clinical diagnosis. . . . Diagnostic roentgenology, especially as it relates to the nervous system, is a primary clinical diagnostic aid in chiropractic and has been since the early 1900's.
>
> In addition, doctors of chiropractic are knowledgeable in the standard and special clinical laboratory procedures and tests usual to modern diagnostic science. . . .
>
> Chiropractic methods are determined by the scope of practice authorized by state law. Essentially, treatment methods include chiropractic manipulation, necessary dietary advice and nutritional supplementation, adjunctive physiotherapeutic and supportive measures, and professional counsel. [46]

This message, which has changed little during multiple editions of the booklet, does not reflect what takes place in the typical chiropractic office. Chiropractors use some of the same tools as their medical "colleagues," but the majority also use questionable procedures. This chapter looks at thermography, leg-length testing, the Toftness device, "electrodiagnostic devices," homeopathy, contour analysis, colonic irrigation, Neural Organization Technique, Bilateral Nasal Specific, and various routine but unproven diagnostic tests. The following chapter focuses on methods related to "nutrition."

Thermography and Its "Ancestors"

Heat-detection has played a significant role in chiropractic's search for its elusive subluxation. A modern chiropractic text on this subject states that D.D. Palmer used the back of his hand to locate "hot boxes" along the spinal column in an effort to detect differences in surface temperature from one side to the other. The authors observed that "this technique, although subjective and unreliable owing to the variable sensitivity of the diagnosing physician, has been taught to chiropractic students since the birth of the profession" [50].

In the mid-1920s, B.J. Palmer became convinced that a "neurocalometer" ("NCM") developed by one of his students could identify the existence, location, and extent of vertebral subluxations. This device consisted of two probes connected to a meter that registered whether points on either side of the spine had different temperatures. B.J. espoused (and insisted upon leasing) the device so vigorously that many of his supporters became alienated, a situation that sociologist Walter I. Wardwell has called "the neurocalometer debacle" [255].

Thermography involves measuring small temperature differences between sides of the body and evaluating the patterns of infrared thermographic images. In the 1960s, thermographic devices attracted medical interest, particularly for screening breast cancer patients, but controlled trials showed that thermography was no more accurate than chance alone. This and subsequent findings have caused most physicians to consider

The Nervo-Scope, one of several NCM descendants, was marketed by a leading chiropractic supply house during the 1970s. Its findings could be charted by connecting it to a recorder. The company's catalog said that the hand-held device "was taking its place alongside the x-ray in importance."

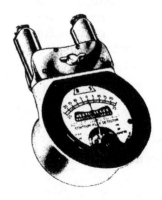

thermography as little more than a potential research tool that should not be used commercially [58]. Both the American Academy of Neurology [4] and the American Academy of Orthopedic Surgeons [198] have issued position papers stating that thermography is unreliable for detecting neurological problems. The recently released report of the Agency for Health Care Policy and Research (see Chapter 12) concluded that thermography is not reliable for assessing patients with acute low-back problems [33:65].

Some chiropractors, however, have embraced thermography and, in 1987, the American Chiropractic Association even set up a group that offers "board certification" [252]. One manufacturer has said its device could "document a patient's progress with each chiropractic adjustment." Another manufacturer has claimed that the pictures produced by its device offer "proof of pain" in cases where x-ray examination shows nothing abnormal. Presumably for this reason, another company has claimed that thermography "increases patient referral from attorneys in personal injury cases." An infrared thermographic examination typically costs hundreds of dollars.

Leg-Length Testing

Many chiropractors tell patients that one leg is shorter than the other. This has been documented by two investigators who visited chiropractors for "checkups." Mark Brown, a reporter for the *Quad-City Times*, a newspaper in Davenport, Iowa, noted in 1981 that on one day during his lengthy investigation, one chiropractor told him his left leg was shorter than his right while another chiropractor told him just the opposite [37]. During 1989, William M. London, Ed.D., assistant professor of health education at Kent State University, visited twenty-three chiropractors in Ohio and Florida who had advertised free consultations or examinations. Of the seventeen who examined him, three said his left leg was shorter than his right leg and two said his right leg was shorter than his left one [21]. In addition, three said he had mild scoliosis and two said he had kyphosis (abnormal rearward curvature of the spine).

The most popular system involving leg-length testing is Activator Methods chiropractic technique, which is taught at chiropractic schools and independent seminars. A 1991 survey by the National Board of Chiropractic Examiners found that 51.2 percent of 4,835 full-time practitioners who responded said they used Activator Methods [49]. The system is based on a premise that "pelvic deficiency"—also called "P.D." or "functional short leg"— is a widespread problem [191]. (This is not an actual or anatomical short leg due to differing lengths of the leg bones.) To diagnose this supposed condition, the practitioner observes the position of the feet with

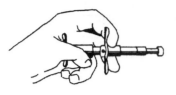

the patient lying facedown on an examining table. The accompanying "spinal imbalances" ("subluxations") are then corrected by applying "adjusting thrusts" with an Activator, a small hand-held, spring-loaded mallet (pictured here) that taps areas of the body considered responsible for the problem [262]. It is not a method of spinal manipulation.

Arlan W. Fuhr, D.C., founder and president of Activator Methods, Inc., has produced a videotape for use in educating patients. During the tape, he explains his methods to a family of four. Using a plastic model of the spine, he states that subluxations of the neck may produce migraine headaches, subluxations of the sixth thoracic vertebra can cause ulcers and shoulder pain, and subluxations of the twelfth thoracic vertebra can produce kidney problems. Activator Methods' 181-page college textbook states that "visual observation will indicate the P.D. side 85% of the time without the doctor even touching the patient" [191]. Sure enough, when the mother lies down on the examining table, Fuhr notes that one of her legs extends past the table about half an inch further than the other leg. After feeling several areas of her spine and zapping supposed problem areas, he repositions her legs (bending them up 90°) and notes that they are the same length. He then repeats these procedures with her head turned to each side and one arm or the other behind her back. Fuhr does not appear to consider that slight variations of hip position or of normal spinal muscle tension are probably responsible for his findings.

Another approach involving leg-length testing is the Morter HealthSystem, developed by M.T. Morter, Jr., of Rogers, Arkansas, a chiropractor who has been president of two chiropractic colleges. One component of the system, Bio Energetic Synchronization Technique (B.E.S.T.) is based on the idea that development and repair of the body are controlled by its electromagnetic field. Its followers postulate that an imbalance in the patient's electromagnetic field causes unequal leg length, which the chiropractor can instantly correct by applying his own electro-magnetic energy to proper points on the body. According to this notion, two fingers on each of the chiropractor's hands are north poles, two are south poles, and the thumbs are electromagnetically neutral. When "imbalance" is detected, the hands are held for a few seconds at "contact points" on the patient's body until "pulsation" is felt and the patient's legs test equally long. Proponents recommend that such testing be started early in infancy and continued at least monthly throughout life.

Morter also teaches that vitality can be maintained "by consuming four times as much alkaline-forming as acid-forming foods." He states that saliva pH [the degree of acidity or alkalinity] should be tested to determine whether symptoms are nutritionally or emotionally based and whether the most effective method of care should be nutritional supplementation and/or adjustive. The supplements include an "alkalizer," an enzyme formula "designed to reduce stress in the body," and a weight-reduction product "designed to alkalize and energize at the same time." The scientific facts, of course, are otherwise. There is no reason to be concerned about the "acidity" or "alkalinity" of either the diet or the body. In the absence of serious disease, digestive and metabolic mechanisms maintain the cells of the body at their appropriate pH regardless of which foods are eaten [25].

Experienced orthopedic physicians, such as Leon Root, M.D., say that leg-length differences rarely cause back pain [205:9]. A few chiropractors have thoroughly examined published literature on leg-length testing and concluded that the procedure is unsubstantiated. In 1992, an extensive review by Donna M. Mannello, D.C., a research associate at Logan College of Chiropractic, concluded that "the available literature does not provide strong evidence of intra- or interexaminer reliability, validity or the clinical significance of these methods" [157]. Do you believe that "functional" difference in leg length is a sign of "subluxation" or an "imbalance" in the body's electromagnetic field?

The Toftness Device

The Toftness Radiation Detector is a hand-held instrument claimed to detect low levels of electromagnetic radiation from the human body and focus it so that a chiropractor could detect conditions requiring treatment. The device, patented in 1971, consists of a plastic cylinder containing a series of plastic lenses. Its inventor, chiropractor Irwing N. Toftness, claimed that energy with a frequency of 69.5 gigahertz emanates from compressed spinal nerves. The device supposedly focused the radiation so the chiropractor could detect it while rubbing his fingers on the detection plate. Rubbing hard could produce a crackling sound similar to that of a Geiger counter. The purported disturbances would then be treated by spinal adjustments.

Yale University's Edmund S. Crelin, Ph.D., who tested the device for the FDA, concluded that it was "hocus-pocus" [60]. He pointed out that

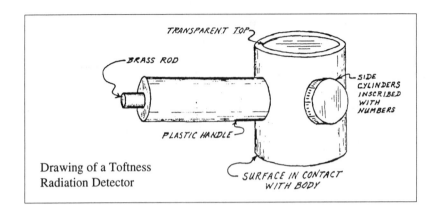

TRANSPARENT TOP

BRASS ROD

SIDE CYLINDERS INSCRIBED WITH NUMBERS

PLASTIC HANDLE

Drawing of a Toftness
Radiation Detector

SURFACE IN CONTACT WITH BODY

radiation at 69.5 gigahertz would penetrate only about one millimeter of body tissue, while the spinal nerves are two to three inches from the body's surface. So even if a dysfunctional nerve could radiate the tiny amount of energy claimed by Toftness, the radiation would be absorbed by surrounding tissues and would not be detectable at or above the body's surface.

In 1984, after winning a lengthy court battle initiated by the FDA, the Justice Department ordered chiropractors who still possessed a Toftness device to return it. The number of chiropractors still using the device is unclear, but 3.3 percent of respondents to the National Board of Chiropractic Examiners' 1991 survey said they used Toftness techniques. And Irwing Toftness is still held in high esteem in many chiropractic circles.

Homeopathy

Homeopathy is based on the unsubstantiated belief that if a large amount of a substance can produce symptoms in a healthy person, infinitesimal amounts can cure illnesses with those symptoms. Homeopathic "remedies" are made from minerals, and various other "natural" substances that are diluted repeatedly. Proponents claim that even if the dilution is so great that no molecule of original substance remains, an "essence" of the active ingredient persists and can stimulate the body's recuperative powers. Critics consider these ideas delusional.

Although homeopathy rates scant mention at most chiropractic schools, the National Board of Chiropractic Examiners' 1991 survey found that 36.9 percent of the respondents listed homeopathy among their treatment techniques. Homeopathy is promoted to chiropractors through articles and ads in their magazines and trade publications. The most active publicist is Frank

J. King, Jr., N.D., D.C., the founder/director of a homeopathic manufacturing company "dedicated to the marriage of homeopathy and chiropractic." In a 1991 interview, King asserted that "homeopathy offers chiropractic the most effective and clinically proven system of correcting sensory nerve interference." His company's *Physician's Reference Manual* advises which of seventy-five products to use for hundreds of symptoms and conditions. King maintains that his formulas are "a valuable adjunct to chiropractic, nutritional supplements, herbals and diets" and can be selected with a "cookbook approach" (using label information), muscle testing (applied kinesiology), an "electroacupuncture" device, leg-length testing (Activator Methods), or even a Toftness device (which was banned by court order in the early 1980s). In an article in the *Digest of Chiropractic Economics*, King presented a case report showing how he had netted $942.96 for eleven treatment visits totaling 107 minutes [134].

Boericke & Tafel, Inc., of Santa Rosa, California, markets six "professional formulas" that "add a new dimension to the practice of chiropractic." A company flyer states that "homeopathy works hand in hand with chiropractic to reinforce the healing process." The company's "clinical guide" booklet lists fifty-five conditions treatable with the six formulas. They include anxiety, disc herniation, scar tissue, frozen shoulder, insomnia, and subluxation.

Professional Health Products Ltd., a Pennsylvania-based company, markets 240 "homeopathic specialties" that include *Angina Drops, Bacterial Immune Stimulator, Cataract Drops, Delirium Formula, Epilepsy Drops, Kidney Stone Drops, Memory Drops, Schizophrenia Drops, Sexual Disorders Formula,* and *Weight Off Drops.*

Federal laws require most drugs to be proven safe and effective, but a loophole has helped homeopathic products escape being held to this standard. The National Council Against Health Fraud regards homeopathic products as "dilute placebos" and believes the FDA should ban them [197]. *Consumer Reports* advises being suspicious of any chiropractor who sells them [47].

"Electrodiagnostic" Devices

A few chiropractors use "electrodiagnostic" devices to help determine what treatment to administer. These devices—also called "electroacupuncture" or Voll devices—are claimed to pinpoint "organ weaknesses" and "food allergies" by detecting "imbalances" in the flow of energy along acupuncture meridians. (Meridians are imaginary channels through which the body's "life force" is alleged to flow.) The devices, which are fancy galvanometers, merely measure the electrical resistance of the patient's skin when touched by a probe. One wire from the device goes to a metal cylinder that the patient holds in one hand. A second wire is connected to a probe, which the operator touches to various points on the patient's other hand or foot. This completes a low-voltage circuit and the device registers the flow of current. The information is then relayed to a gauge or computer screen that provides a numerical readout. The size of the number actually depends on how hard the probe is pressed against the patient's skin [25]. The treatment selected may include homeopathic remedies, acupuncture, dietary change, vitamin supplements, and/or spinal adjustments.

One such device, pictured here, is said to help determine the "bioenergetic compatibility" of homeopathic formulas and nutritional supple-

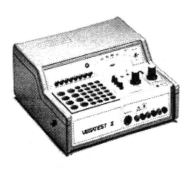

ments. This is done by inserting ampules of various test substances into a metal block that is plugged into the circuit between the patient and the device. The substances supposedly "resonate with various bioenergetic weaknesses, interferences, and imbalances." The findings are then used to prescribe nutritional products and homeopathic remedies. A flyer for the device states that it is illegal to represent that it is useful in the prevention, diagnosis, and treatment of any disease or condition. Why else do you suppose any chiropractor would use it?

Contour Analysis

Contour analysis, also called moire contourography, is a procedure in which an angled light is passed through a grid to the surface of the patient's body to produce a moire effect that is photographed [235]. The resultant picture resembles a topographic map; the greater the number of concentric lines, the greater the elevation from the furthest part of the body. Reproducible results can be obtained if the patient is positioned carefully, but even slight shifts in position alter the patterns. However, as

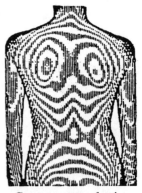

Contour analysis photograph from a yellow pages ad that offers free screening.

noted in the Mercy Conference report: "the results are difficult to quantify and no good correlation to physical findings exists. Adequate interpretation is therefore lacking" [97]. The conference report, described in Chapter 15, reflects a consensus of chiropractic leaders on the validity of most methods used by chiropractors.

Claims made by users and manufacturers of contour-analysis devices range from wishful thinking to complete bunkum. Many chiropractors claim that moire patterns provide valuable information to detect "spinal faults" and measure the progress of their treatment. The marketer of one device claims that the procedure: "reveals distortions, fixations, pronations, muscle imbalance, muscle spasms, anomalies, spinal dynamics"; enables chiropractors to "know where and when to treat . . . when NOT to treat"; and provides "before-and-after proof of treatment." An article used to promote this device states that contourography can "reveal distortions . . . that could irritate spinal nerves and interrupt the flow of energy along [acupuncture] meridians." Another article claims that the device produces "stress patterns [that] resemble fingerprints and are just as individual and revealing to the chiropractor as fingerprints are to an FBI agent."

The more prudent view is that contourography is a marketing gimmick which enables chiropractors to attract patients and boost their income. Patterns that depart from the "ideal" are easily produced by positioning the patient poorly. After treatment, correction of these "abnormalities" can be demonstrated with another examination in which the patient is appropriately positioned.

Colonic Irrigation

Colonic irrigation, also called colonic lavage, is based on the incorrect theory that food in the intestines may rot and form toxins that are absorbed and poison the entire body. Some proponents claim to wash out "toxins" that cause fatigue, headache, insomnia, depression, and many other problems. However, no such toxins have ever been identified. Some proponents make unsubstantiated claims that "toxic bowel settlement" is washed out or that parasitic infestations can be eliminated in this manner. The scientific community gave credence to the concept of autointoxication around the turn of the century but discarded it as worthless during the 1930s. Nevertheless, three editions of the American Chiropractic Association's *Basic Chiropractic Procedural Manual* issued from 1977 through 1984 contain this bizarre advice:

Physicians, particularly those dealing with many emotional disorders, encounter a large number of cases of constipation, autointoxication, and high blood pressure, with such acute symptoms as vertigo, nausea, headache, irritability, insomnia, and excitement, which are due to neglect of colon hygiene. The cleansing enema affords the quickest relief of several of the acute symptoms. . . .

[Colonic irrigation] is particularly indicated in involution melancholia, psychoses with cerebral arteriosclerosis, psychoses with epilepsy, and neurasthenia. In order to obtain the relief of autointoxication and avoid elevating the blood pressure, the treatment must be managed very carefully. Massage, fomentations, vibrassage, or sinusoidal current are sometimes applied with or following the colonic flushing. [211]

Colonic irrigation is done by inserting a tube up to a foot or more into the rectum and flowing up to twenty gallons of warm water in and out. Usually a series of enemas is given, which can induce or worsen constipation. Some practitioners add coffee to the enema. The large amounts of caffeine absorbed are likely to cause nervousness. More seriously, the large amount of fluid can cause electrolytic imbalance by potassium depletion, producing illness or even death [71]. Improper sanitation of the instruments used in the process caused an outbreak of amebiasis in Colorado, when microbes from one person's intestine were transferred to numerous other patients [38:169]. Surgery for perforation of the bowel was required in ten of these cases, and seven persons died. Deaths from other complications, such as a ruptured appendix, have been reported.

In 1988, 2 percent of about 2,400 respondents to a survey by *Dynamic Chiropractic* (the leading chiropractic newspaper) said they used colonic irrigation in their practices [110].

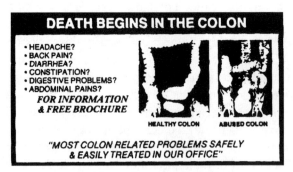

Solicitation from a chiropractor who recommends colonic irrigation.

Treatment or Torture?

Although Neural Organization Technique (NOT) and Bilateral Nasal Specific (BNS) are not widely used, they deserve mention because they are often directed at handicapped children.

NOT, an offshoot of "applied kinesiology" and various "cranial techniques," includes the notion that the skull is an "extension of the spine" [75]. NOT's proponents claim that "blocked neural pathways" caused by misaligned skull bones can cause learning disorders, cerebral palsy, schizophrenia, Down's syndrome, colorblindness, bedwetting, nightmares, and various other problems. Its practitioners claim that "adjusting" these bones by applying pressure to various structures of the head can cure these problems. (This claim is not only unsubstantiated but defies medical knowledge that the bones of the skull are fused tightly by age two.) NOT's originator, Carl A. Ferreri, D.C., of New York City, says he has trained hundreds of chiropractors in the use of his techniques.

NOT came to public attention in 1988 when chiropractors subjected children to it in a "research" program sponsored by school officials in Del Norte County, California. For five months, dozens of children from age four to sixteen, with epilepsy, Down's syndrome, cerebral palsy, dyslexia, and various other learning disorders, were "treated" by having their skull compressed with viselike hand pressure. The children were also forced to endure painful thumb pressure against the roof of the mouth and finger pressure against their eyes. According to news reports, the children struggled, cried, and screamed as they were forcibly restrained. One reportedly experienced his first seizure when his eye sockets were "adjusted." Some of the children became violent, explosive, rebellious, uncontrollable, and lacking in self-motivation and drive [56] [249]. In 1991, a jury ordered Ferreri to pay $565,000 in damages to seven children and their parents who had filed suit for physical and emotional pain related to the treatment. Two other chiropractors involved in the case settled out of court for a total of $207,000.

Bilateral Nasal Specific is another cranial technique in which a finger cot is pushed as far as possible into each side of the nose and inflated. According to proponents, this procedure aids circulation to the brain and provides it with better nutrition. Its developer claims that BNS can cure mental retardation in children, make dwarfs grow taller, and straighten out the heads of babies after birth. The treatment, in addition to being painful, is not risk-free. In 1983, a Canadian baby was asphyxiated after the finger cot slipped off the syringe on which it was mounted and lodged in the child's windpipe. The practitioner was found guilty of manslaughter, fined $1,000, and ordered to stop using BNS. A 1985 report stated that about two hundred chiropractors had been using BNS [150].

Unproven Routine Diagnostics

Besides the obviously pseudoscientific nonsense described above, chiropractors use many diagnostic techniques that have never been scientifically demonstrated to be reliable or clinically significant. In recent years, qualified researchers on the faculty of chiropractic colleges have evaluated many of the profession's popular techniques. So far, most published reports have concluded that whatever technique was considered had not been proven reliable, reproducible, and/or clinically significant. In 1991, for example, after reviewing forty-five articles concerning the reliability of numerous routine chiropractic diagnostic tests, Mitchell Haas, D.C., reported:

> Only 10 studies . . . have properly supported conclusions, while an additional three studies contained correct conclusions by coincidence. Eight investigations had invalid designs and three contained claims that were contradicted by the author's findings. Half the studies . . . have conclusions that were based on inappropriate or inconclusive statistical analysis. To date, the research presented in the chiropractic literature cannot substantiate claims concerning the reliability of any diagnostic instrumentation or palpatory procedures commonly employed by chiropractic physicians. [93]

The procedures Haas reviewed included x-ray diagnosis, leg-length measurement, static palpation, range of motion and posture evaluation, thermography, infrared detectors, muscle testing, and several other procedures. Haas concluded that based on chiropractic literature, claims of reliability for any of these tests were "premature." He then admonished journal editors to protect "the statistically uninformed" by rejecting manuscripts based on low-quality research.

In the late 1980s, Joseph C. Keating, Ph.D., and three associates conducted a controlled trial designed to see whether chiropractors using common diagnostic techniques would have similar findings. Simply inspecting the designated areas of the patient's spine or feeling whether they were warm or tender provided somewhat consistent results, but there was little significant agreement for four other techniques (active and passive motion palpation, muscle tension palpation and misalignment palpation) [131]. Keating added that even when different chiropractic examiners can detect the same findings in a patient, this "says nothing about the clinical usefulness, meaning or validity of the examination procedure."

In a subsequent literature review, David M. Panzer, D.C., concluded that motion palpation (a technique purported to detect abnormalities in joint mobility), though widely practiced, had not yet been vindicated in that (1) most studies have demonstrated marginal-to-poor interexaminer reliability, (2) the abnormalities found by motion palpation have not been shown to relate to underlying motion abnormalities, and (3) the underlying movement abnormalities have not been shown to be associated with pathological changes or articular derangements, but may just be normal variants [183].

In yet another critique, Karel Lewit (a physician) and Craig Liebenson, D.C., discussed various procedures chiropractors use to diagnose problems and evaluate their patients' progress. They concluded that "there is an urgent need for research in palpation, which could provide basic scientific credibility to manipulative techniques." They also noted that "the historic as well as rational importance of palpation . . . is not sufficient to uphold its credibility in the managed care environment of the future. Research into the nature of palpation is needed to legitimize this crucial part of the chiropractic art" [146]. This is a gentle way of saying that this fundamental chiropractic procedure cannot withstand scientific scrutiny.

Inappropriate X-ray Procedures

Despite the fact that the use of x-rays should be based on clinical findings, many chiropractors perform x-ray examinations as a routine screening procedure. In fact, many believe that virtually every patient who enters their office should be x-rayed to look for "subluxations." *Consumer Reports* has labeled this practice as "twice removed from reality" because "it depends upon an unscientific appraisal of a nonexistent disease" [48]. Yet a 1993 survey of chiropractic colleges found that several still taught that subluxations can be identified on x-ray films (see Chapter 4) [261].

Besides purporting to find imaginary subluxations of doubtful clinical significance, chiropractors use x-rays for other purposes for which the diagnostic tool has not been validated. Reed B. Phillips, D.C., Ph.D., a former president of the American Chiropractic Board of Roentgenology Examining Board, has observed:

> The chiropractic physician justifies the use of x-ray in the manage-
> ment of low back pain to a) rule out pathology, b) perform a
> biomechanical evaluation, c) protect against medicolegal action, d)
> obtain financial gain and e) out of habit. The literature fails to
> support or justify the use of x-ray in the management of acute low
> back pain for any of the above listed reasons. [192]

In a recent interview, Phillips, who now is president of Los Angeles College
of Chiropractic, said that studies provide no support for the use of x-rays for
most cases of low-back pain. If an injury is serious enough to require x-ray
evaluation (if there are symptoms such as shooting pains or numbness in the
legs, for example), the patient should be referred to a physician [259].

Many other knowledgeable chiropractors have criticized the indiscriminate use of x-rays. The Mercy Guidelines state that the need for x-ray
examination should be based on the patient's history and physical findings
and that the potential benefits should be weighed against the risks of
exposure to ionizing radiation. The guidelines also state that "routine"
radiographic screening is inappropriate and full-spine films are not appropriate for routine evaluations or reevaluations except in cases of scoliosis
[97:14]. Ted Fickel, D.C., Ph.D., who has taught at two chiropractic
colleges and has a doctoral degree in biomedical sciences, has stated that
diagnostic x-rays should not be obtained unless bony injury or other
pathology is suspected and that bony pathologies other than cancer are
usually accompanied by obvious signs and symptoms [76] [77]. He has also
explained why screening elderly people to detect degenerative changes is
unlikely to be fruitful:

> Degenerative changes occur in asymptomatic cervical and lumbar
> spines with increasing frequency in middle age and beyond.... The
> assumption that the presence of these degenerative findings ex-
> plains musculoskeletal complaints is unfounded because these
> changes are found with approximately equal frequency in symp-
> tomatic and asymptomatic patients. [76]

As noted in Chapter 5, some chiropractors provide "free x-rays" as a
marketing technique. These chiropractors usually find "subluxations," for
which they propose long courses of "treatment." In 1967, the American
Chiropractic Association "strongly condemned as unethical and dangerous
the practice of advertising free spinal x-ray examinations and other indiscriminate uses of x-ray as part of practice building schemes and/or for other
equally unethical purposes." In 1993, this resolution was reworded:

> Resolved, that the American Chiropractic Association strongly

condemn as unethical and potentially dangerous, the advertising of free x-rays, or indiscriminate use of x-rays, without an accompanying statement that: to avoid needless health hazards associated with ionizing radiation, no such free x-rays (or other indiscriminate use of x-rays) shall be undertaken unless there is prior demonstrated clinical need.

Many chiropractors attribute clinical significance to trivial x-ray findings and consider these justification for x-raying every patient. This viewpoint has been justifiably criticized by both medical and chiropractic authorities. Lewit, for example, has concluded that spinal asymmetry is the rule, not the exception, and that this is of dubious clinical significance [145:45]. Neurologist Scott Haldeman, D.C., M.D., Ph.D., has stated that minor misalignments of vertebrae "are normal and not necessarily a sign of trouble" [47]. Daniel Futch, D.C., executive director of the National Association for Chiropractic Medicine agrees that minute vertebral irregularities "show up on almost anyone's x-ray," but alone have no effect on health [81].

During the late 1980s, surveys done by the FDA Center for Devices and Radiological Health found that chiropractors were more likely than other practitioners to perform their spinal x-ray examinations improperly [208]. The study found that 69 (48 percent) of 143 chiropractors were underprocessing their films improperly, which meant that to obtain the same quality picture they would have to expose patients to larger amounts of radiation. The corresponding figures were 33 percent for hospitals, 25 percent for radiologists in private practice, and 35 percent for nonradiologist private practitioners.

One last dubious technique used by many chiropractors is the calculation of vertebral offsetting based on x-ray findings. Haas's review of the chiropractic literature on the interexaminer reliability of these x-ray marking and diagnostic techniques found "contradictory results" and "findings that have not been fully substantiated" [93]. According to Peter J. Modde, D.C., this method of measuring supposed spinal subluxations "appears very sophisticated to those unschooled in spinal dynamics. Nevertheless, in my opinion it has no basis in fact" [164:245]. In an article in *Medical Economics* magazine, reformist Mark Sanders, D.C., put the matter more bluntly:

D.C.s employ a variety of elaborate x-ray marking systems and techniques to determine misalignments and make therapeutic choices. I know of no documentation supporting the validity of these systems, but here's a description of a commonly used technique: The practitioner takes a full spinal x-ray, compares it with an idealized version of the spine, then measures how much the patient's vertebrae deviate from the ideal. After tallying the deviations—let's say the total is 30 millimeters—the chiropractor determines the number of spinal manipulations the patient is supposed to receive: 30. To me, this lacks a rational basis, since there's little evidence that slight postural distortions are correlated with back pain. The literature isn't even clear on what the "perfect" spine looks like. [209]

Phillips also minces no words. He states: "Failure to adequately support and justify the use of x-ray for biomechanical evaluation as an integral part of patient care borders on abdication of the right to take x-rays" [192].

The Bottom Line

Craig F. Nelson, D.C., an associate professor at Northwestern College, has provided an interesting insight into the chiropractic marketplace:

One of the most distinctive features of chiropractic is that it supports dozens of different techniques, most of which purport to accomplish the same thing: evaluate (diagnose) the structural status of the human frame, particularly the vertebral column, and prescribe corrective procedures.

The various chiropractic techniques . . . usually come complete with a theoretical framework [and claim] a unique relationship with the truth. . . . Different techniques with different theoretical bases may in fact lead to similar treatment regimens. But it is also true that many of these techniques are truly distinct and incompatible with each other. . . .

There is no comparable circumstance in any other health care profession. [169]

Nelson certainly is correct. With most of the basic diagnostic methods of chiropractic still not validated and the widespread use of methods that *cannot* be validated, it isn't hard to understand why chiropractic has contributed almost nothing to the advancement of health science.

8

Nutrition-Related Nonsense

Chiropractors represent themselves as "drugless practitioners." Indeed, they are not legally permitted to prescribe drugs. Some go so far as to advise that the use of medically prescribed drugs is "unnatural" and counterproductive. The American Chiropractic Association's public education materials have included messages like "Beware of overuse of drugs," "Don't be a pill popper," and "Chiropractic care protects your health without drugs!" The World Chiropractic Alliance (an organization for "straight" chiropractors) urges patients to just "say no to all drugs." Tragic examples have been reported of patients with diabetes, epilepsy, high blood pressure, and other serious diseases who suffered complications or even died as a result of abandoning effective pharmacologic treatment.

Instead of drugs, what do chiropractors offer? Many sell supplement products in their offices, usually for at least twice their wholesale cost. A typical regimen can cost several dollars per day. The offerings include vitamins, minerals, amino acids, dehydrated vegetables, other food-related substances, freeze-dried animal tissue, enzymes, herbs, and many combinations of these substances. *Consumer Reports* once remarked that these products enable chiropractors to "prescribe" something [79]. This chapter scrutinizes some of these products and how chiropractors decide which to recommend.

What Chiropractors "Prescribe"

Chiropractic suppliers are marketing thousands of pills and potions

97

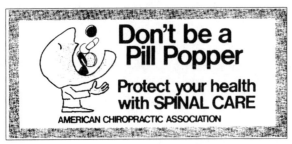 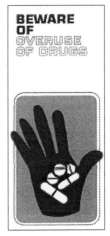

Billboard poster and flyer distributed in the 1970s by the American Chiropractic Association. The pamphlet listed side effects of antibiotics and other valuable drugs and said nothing about their benefits. The poster and other "pill popper" materials are still available from the ACA.

intended for therapeutic use. Some are available through health-food stores, while others are marketed primarily or exclusively through chiropractors. Some products are intended to prevent or treat nutrient deficiencies (which, as noted below, may not actually be a problem). Some products are claimed to "strengthen the immune system," "balance the body's chemistry," or furnish "nutritional support" to various body organs. Others are claimed to be effective against various diseases. Chiropractors learn about them from product literature, seminars, exhibits at chiropractic conventions, and material provided by "independent" regional distributors. Some manufacturers provide copies of articles from the popular press or health-food magazines that mention substances contained in their products. A few companies have distributed elaborate manuals listing diseases their products can supposedly treat. Other companies stress quality or price advantage and let the chiropractors figure out for themselves what the products are for.

Many products are simply named after a body part, organ, or organ system (e.g., *Nutra-Disc, Ora-Brain, Neuroplex*); bodily function (*Anabolic MegaPak, Gluco-Stabil*); or health problem (*ArthEase*). The ones named after organs usually contain bits of freeze-dried tissue from one or more animal organs and are not supposed to contain active hormones. Called "glandulars," these products are claimed to "support," "strengthen," or "rejuvenate" the corresponding body parts. These claims, however, have no scientific basis.

Oral enzymes that are claimed to enhance metabolic processes are a similar rip-off. Enzymes are proteins. Within the human body, enzymes act as catalysts for bodily reactions. The enzymes in foods, however, are not absorbed intact into the body. When consumed, like other proteins, they are digested into smaller constituents. Even if they were absorbed, enzymes for plants would not catalyze the metabolic processes of humans.

The most fanciful product involving animal tissue and "enzymes" is probably *Spine Align*, which, according to its manufacturer, can (1) help repair, regenerate, correct, and normalize the spine; (2) help, support, and strengthen chiropractic adjustments; and (3) "activate the body's own Innate." Its ingredients, listed on the label below, include "whole spinal column" (from cows) and "homeopathically prepared" gold. Its processing is said to preserve "biologically active substances" that occur naturally in the animal tissue from which the product is prepared. The manufacturer, Vita-Herbs Inc., of St. Louis, also markets *AdrenaAid, Juvenation, LVR,* and *Thymamune.*

Another remarkable conception is *Chiro-Zyme*, a line of "carefully formulated combinations of herbs, vitamins and minerals with plant enzymes targeted to organs stressed by subluxation." Twenty-four of the products in its 1995 catalog are named with an abbreviation for spinal segments and an organ or body function. *C8 to T1 Thy*, for example, is said to "nourish the tissues of the thyroid gland stressed by subluxations of the upper thoracic and cervical spine," while *T1 to T7 Rsp* is for "tissues of the respiratory system stressed by subluxations of the upper and mid-thoracic spine."

Many products are marketed to chiropractors with literature that contains double-talk. PhysioLogics, of Boulder, Colorado, for example, markets formulas "designed for and sold exclusively to Health Care

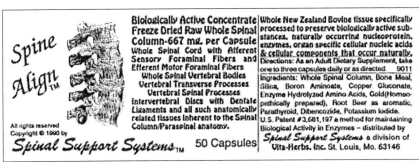

Label from bottle of *Spine Align*, a product marketed with the claim that "organ specific cellular components help repair, regenerate, correct and normalize the specific cellular complexes they were derived from."

Professionals for dispensing in clinics and offices under professional supervision." Its catalog states that the products "are not intended to diagnose, treat, cure, or prevent any disease." Yet the products include: *Paraclear* ("a combination of 17 . . . ingredients that work synergistically to support the body's natural defense system function against parasites"); *Thyroid Support Formula* ("supports healthy thyroid function" and "offers dietary assistance to combat exhaustion and mental fatigue"); and *VitaCardia* ("nutritionally supports the cardiovascular

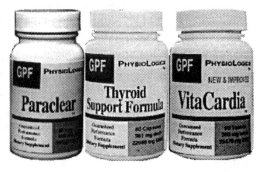

system" and "provides nutrients . . . essential to the maintenance of healthy blood pressure").

The percentage of chiropractors engaging in unscientific nutrition practices is unknown, but several reports suggest that it is substantial. In 1988, 74 percent of about 2,400 respondents to a survey by *Dynamic Chiropractic* (the leading chiropractic newspaper) reported using nutrition supplements in their practices [110]. In 1991, 83.5 percent of 4,835 full-time practitioners who responded to a survey by the National Board of Chiropractic Examiners (NBCE) said they had used "nutritional counseling, therapy or supplements" within the previous two years [49]. *Consumer Reports* estimated that at least 150 supplement companies market through chiropractors [47]. Some chiropractors charge thousands of dollars for programs involving "diagnostic" evaluations, supplements, adjustments, and/or massage over a period of several months [25].

Muscle-Testing Systems

Many chiropractors prescribe supplements as part of an "alternative" approach to diagnosis and treatment. The most common of these is applied kinesiology (AK), a pseudoscientific system of muscle-testing and therapy based on assertions that specific muscle weaknesses are signs of disease in body organs. Finding a "weak" muscle supposedly enables the chiropractor to pinpoint illness in the corresponding internal organs in the body. For example, a weak muscle in the chest might indicate a liver problem, and a weak muscle near the groin might indicate "adrenal insufficiency." While subjecting the patient to various substances—usually foods or vitamins placed in the mouth—the chiropractor tests the strength of various muscles. If a muscle tests "weaker" after a substance is placed in the patient's mouth, it supposedly signifies disease in the organ associated with that muscle. If the muscle tests "stronger," the substance supposedly can remedy problems in the corresponding body parts. Some practitioners contend that muscle-testing can also help diagnose nutritional deficiencies, allergies, and other adverse reactions to foods. According to this theory, when a muscle tests "weak," the provocative substance is bad for the patient. Treatment usually involves nutritional supplements, special diets, and spinal manipulation.

These notions are far removed from reality, but some chiropractors carry them even further. Some perform their tests with the test substance held in the patient's hand or touching a surface of the patient's body. Some perform "surrogate testing" in which a parent is tested while holding or touching the child and the findings are considered applicable to the child!

AK was initiated in 1964 by George J. Goodheart, Jr., and has become quite elaborate. Goodheart claims that AK techniques can also be used to evaluate nerve, vascular, and lymphatic systems; the body's nutritional state; the flow of "energy" along "acupuncture meridians"; and "cerebro spinal fluid function." The seventy-page chapter on "meridian therapy" in a leading AK textbook advises that subluxations influence the status of meridian system and vice versa [254]. The NBCE's 1991 survey found that 37.2 percent of those who responded said they used AK in their practice,

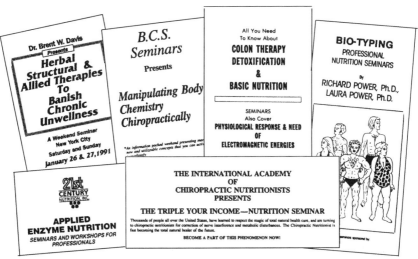

Brochures from nutrition-related seminars offered to chiropractors during the past twenty years.

65.5 percent said they used acupressure/meridian therapy, and 11.8 percent said they used acupuncture [49].

The International College of Applied Kinesiology (ICAK) has set "standards" based on the work of Goodheart and his followers. "Certification" by its board (which is not recognized by chiropractic's official accrediting body) requires a minimum of three hundred hours of study under an ICAK diplomate, five thousand hours of practical experience, authorship of two research papers, and passage of written and practical examinations.

Competent researchers have subjected muscle-testing procedures to several well-designed tests and demonstrated what should be obvious to rational persons. Some have found no difference in muscle response from one substance to another, while others have found no difference between the results with test substances and with placebos. One study, for example, found that the diagnosis of nutritional deficiencies did not correspond to blood serum analysis [133]. Another found no effect from administering the nutrients "expected" to strengthen a muscle diagnosed as "weak" by AK practitioners [247]. A review of twenty research papers published by ICAK concluded that because "none of the papers included adequate statistical analyses, no valid conclusions could be drawn from their findings" [137]. Researchers who conducted an elaborate double-blind trial concluded that "muscle response appeared to be a random phenomenon" [94].

ICAK attempts to defend its cherished notions by stating that muscle-testing should be used as a diagnostic aid rather than the sole basis for diagnosis and that many muscle-testers are not practicing true AK. The fact is, however, that *all* of it is absurd.

Contact Reflex Analysis

Contact Reflex Analysis (CRA) is an elaborate pseudoscientific system that resembles aspects of applied kinesiology. Its codeveloper and leading proponent is Dick A. Versendaal, D.C., of Holland, Michigan. Versendaal claims that CRA can "test every conceivable condition in the human body . . . help that patient, and know how long it will take for that patient to get well." Testing is done by pulling on the patient's outstretched arm while placing one's finger or hand on one of about seventy-five "reflex" points on the patient's body. (Versendaal states that the front of the hand is electrically "positive," the back is "negative," and the fingers are "neutral.") If the arm is weak and can be pulled downward, the reflex "blows," indicating that disease corresponding to the reflex is present [251]. To correct the alleged problems, large numbers of nutritional supplements are prescribed, typically at a cost of several dollars a day. Most of these are pills made from dehydrated vegetables and animal organs. A chiropractor/naturopath who is "chief medical consultant" to a homeopathic manufacturer says he uses CRA to determine which homeopathic remedies to use.

Versendaal's teachings are filled with bizarre notions that conflict with what is known about human anatomy, physiology, and disease. Yet his seminars are sponsored by a chiropractic college. Videotapes of the seminars show him diagnosing "diseases" in parts of the body that he neither touches nor examines. In one patient he diagnoses an "ankle subluxation" by testing a "reflex point" on the patient's chest!

NUTRI-SPEC

NUTRI-SPEC, which stands for "Nutritional Specificity Through Scientific Testing," is the brainchild of Guy R. Schenker, D.C., of Mifflintown, Pennsylvania. It has been promoted for several years through full-page ads in the *Digest of Chiropractic Economics*. A flyer for NUTRI-SPEC claims that it gives the chiropractor a "scientific testing system to determine the specific nutrition needs of every patient in your own office in 5 minutes; and the supplements to meet those needs." The determinations are based on the patient's respiratory rate, body temperature, blood pressure, pulse, breath-holding ability, pupil size, degree of thickness or coating of the tongue, saliva and urine characteristics, and abdominal reflexes.

Using NUTRI-SPEC's unique scoring system, the chiropractor then decides whether the patient is in or out of "water/electrolyte balance," "anaerobic/dysaerobic balance," "acid/alkaline balance," and "sympathetic/parasympathetic balance." The test findings also enable the chiropractor to diagnose "sex hormone insufficiency," "myocardial insufficiency," "pineal stress," "thymus stress," and about twenty-five other fanciful conditions. The "imbalances" are corrected with dietary measures, "oxygenic" supplements, and mineral products purchased from the chiropractor, who obtains them from Schenker's company.

Iridology

Iridology is yet another pseudoscientific diagnosis-and-treatment system based on the notion that all disease is registered in the eye. Practitioners, many of whom are chiropractors, claim that specific parts of the iris (the colored portion of the eye surrounding the pupil) reflect the status of each organ of the body. Scores of charts alleging such relationships have been published, but the differences in the location and interpretation of their iris signs vary considerably. Iridologists claim that states of health and disease can be diagnosed according to the color, texture, and location of various pigment flecks in the eye. They also purport to diagnose "imbalances" and treat them with vitamins, minerals, herbs, and similar products.

Bernard Jensen, D.C., the leading American iridologist, states that "Nature has provided us with a miniature television screen showing the most remote portions of the body by way of nerve reflex responses" [124]. However, there is no reliable evidence suggesting that areas of the iris "correspond" with other parts of the body.

Though attractive due to its simplicity and mystique, iridology has been scientifically discredited as a diagnostic system. The anatomical facts preclude its published claims. According to optometrist Russell S. Worrall, the iris is not an extension of the brain, the optic nerve is not connected to the iris, and, despite great research on the eye's neural pathways, there is no evidence of any nerve connection between the body and the iris [269]. In fact, a scientific evaluation of iridology published in 1979 found that Jensen and two other practitioners could not determine the presence or absence of kidney disease among patients, one-third of whom had such disease [230]. The study's authors also warned that serious harm could result from a false diagnosis of serious disease or a missed diagnosis of a real disease. A similar test of Dutch iridologists published in 1988 found that they could not distinguish patients with gallstones from healthy control patients [138]. Gallbladder disease was chosen because the iridologists themselves had said it was "easy to see."

The National Council Against Health Fraud's position paper on chiropractic suggests that iridologists use a method similar to "cold reading" by fortune-tellers:

> Using a chart as a guide, the clinician fishes for past and present health problems. The subject may be quizzed, "have you had problems with your stomach, liver, back, etc.?" If the patient acknowledges that he/she has, or ever has had, any kind of problem in the area in question, a "hit" is claimed and the "finding" is exploited. If the chart indicates a problem that the subject does not acknowledge, it can be claimed that there is "a weakness and a tendency for disease in the area" (a finding which opens the door for "preventive" treatments to keep the alleged disease from occurring). Thus the practitioner is never judged as wrong. [196]

All sorts of misdiagnoses, from the humorous to the terrifying, have been reported. An investigative reporter who was a vegetarian, for example, was told that she probably ate too much meat. An accountant with heart disease was misdiagnosed as having cancer, which caused great unnecessary mental anguish until reason prevailed.

Hair Analysis

Many chiropractors use hair analysis as a basis for prescribing nutritional supplements. The test is administered by sending a hair sample, usually from the back of the patient's neck, to a commercial laboratory for measurement of its mineral content. The lab then issues a computerized printout that indicates mineral "deficiencies" or "excesses." The test usually costs from $25 to $60. Although hair analysis has limited value as

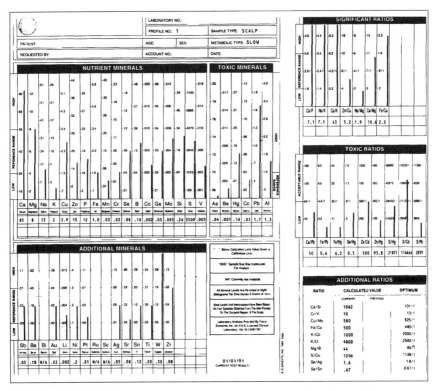

The typical hair analysis report includes a myriad of numbers. This one includes values for thirty-six minerals, "significant ratios," "toxic ratios," and "additional ratios." Versions are available with "comprehensive interpretations" for both chiropractor and patient.

a screening device for exposure to lead and other heavy metals, it is *not* reliable for evaluating the nutritional status of individuals. In 1983 and 1984, Dr. Stephen Barrett sent hair samples from two healthy teenage girls to thirteen commercial hair analysis laboratories. Each lab received two identical samples from each girl, three weeks apart, under different assumed names. Barrett concluded that even if hair analysis were a valuable diagnostic tool, most of the labs were not reliable:

> The reported levels of most minerals varied considerably between identical samples sent to the same laboratory and from laboratory to laboratory. The laboratories disagreed about what was "normal" or "usual" for many of the minerals. Most reports contained computerized interpretations that were voluminous, bizarre, and potentially frightening to patients. Six laboratories recommended food supplements, but the types and amounts varied widely from report to report and from laboratory to laboratory. Literature from most of the laboratories suggested that their reports were useful in managing a wide variety of diseases and supposed nutritional imbalances. However, hair analysis used in this manner is unscientific, economically wasteful, and probably illegal. [16]

Many chiropractic leaders have also criticized the procedure via the Mercy Consensus Conference report (see Chapter 15). The report states that hair analysis may have experimental usefulness but is "not indicated for screening of nutritional status" in symptom-free individuals or for "the determination of nutritional imbalances" [97:73]. In other words, chiropractors should not be using it in day-to-day practice.

Amino Acid Analysis

Proponents claim that amino acid analysis of blood and/or urine is useful in uncovering a wide range of nutritional and metabolic disorders. As with hair analysis, the test report may be accompanied by a lengthy computer print-out containing speculations about the patient's state of health. These claims are false. Like hair analysis, amino acid analysis is not valid for determining the body's nutritional or metabolic state or for "prescribing" nutritional supplements.

Essential Metabolics Analysis (EMA)

SpectraCell Laboratories, Inc., of Houston, Texas, claims that the majority of Americans have nutrient deficiencies and that "intracellular nutrient deficiencies" even occur in over 40 percent of the more than one hundred million Americans taking multivitamins as "insurance." Furthermore, according to a company flyer:

> Today, there is a scientific way to precisely measure your nutrient status. It's a personal nutrient analysis called Essential Metabolics Analysis (EMA) and it's available only from SpectraCell Laboratories. The EMA is like a window on your cells, allowing your physician to look inside and identify individual nutrient needs. A targeted, tailored plan of dietary changes or supplements can then be prescribed with confidence.

Many ads from SpectraCell Laboratories have appeared in periodicals published for chiropractors. The company's information packet states that the test is performed by placing lymphocytes (a type of white blood cell) from the patient's blood into petri dishes containing various concentrations of nutrients. A growth stimulant is added and, a few days later, technicians identify the dishes in which "greatest cell growth" takes place, which supposedly points to a deficiency. The test costs $325.

Company literature states that 90 percent of patients tested are "functionally deficient" and that patients with arthritis, cancer, cardiovascular disease, chronic fatigue, diabetes, immune disorders, multiple sclerosis, obesity, and several other health problems "can benefit from the SpectraCell's EMA, since these conditions are directly or indirectly linked to nutrient deficiencies." But Victor Herbert, M.D., J.D., who helped develop the use of lymphocyte cultures to diagnose nutrient deficiency, regards EMA as a supplement-promoting gimmick:

> Properly performed lymphocyte cultures have a legitimate role in testing for certain nutrient deficiencies. But they are not appropriate for general screening or for diagnosing "nutrient deficiencies" in the manner used by EMA. . . . The EMA test merely reflects the size of nutrient storage in lymphocytes (amounts greater than are needed for normal cellular function). . . . Low storage, which the test reports, is not the same thing as deficiency and is often found in normal people. [25]

Live Cell Analysis

Live cell analysis is carried out by examining blood with a dark-field microscope to which a television monitor has been attached. Both practitioner and patient can then see the blood cells, which appear as dark bodies outlined in white. The practitioner may make a videotape or take polaroid photographs of the television picture for himself and the patient, and the results are used as a basis for prescribing costly vitamin supplements. Dark-field microscopy and videomicroscopy are valid scientific tools, but live cell analysis involves misinterpreting the significance of blood cell characteristics and artifacts that occur as the blood sample dries. James Lowell, Ph.D., who investigated the procedure in 1986, concluded that it was "high-tech hokum" that probably was used by a few hundred practitioners, some of whom were not chiropractors [151]. The number of chiropractors using it today is unknown.

Misuse of Computerized Blood Chemistry Analysis

Since 1984, two medical doctors in Colorado have marketed a computerized evaluation called Nutrabalance, which offers chiropractors and other health professionals a "comprehensive nutritional program" to "improve . . . patient care and . . . profitability." The evaluation is based on the results of a blood chemistry profile and a urinalysis performed at a legitimate laboratory and submitted to Nutrabalance for interpretation. Nutrabalance then issues a lengthy computerized report which classifies the patient according to fourteen "metabolic types," lists supposed health problem areas, and recommends dietary changes and food supplements from a manufacturer chosen by the patient's doctor. The process is similar to hair analysis schemes except that, unlike the hair tests, the blood and urine tests are legitimate. The metabolic types—most of which are named after a gland or other body organ—do not correspond to anything known to medical science, and the supplement recommendations are nutritionally senseless. The interpretation of the tests is also improper. Medical laboratories list a normal "clinical range" for each laboratory value they report. Nutrabalance uses a narrower "physiologic range," which means that some normal lab values will be classified as abnormal.

Recently, an official of the American Chiropractic Association Council on Nutrition recommended a simpler "computerized blood chemistry analysis" for use in chiropractic offices. About forty blood test results are entered into a computer, which compares each laboratory value with the average for that value and reports on the significance of each "deviated lab result . . . based on body physiology at the molecular tissue and organ level." The five-page report also suggests which supplement products will correct the alleged "deviations."

When properly interpreted, blood chemistry screening tests and urinalysis can provide useful information about a person's health status. Since most abnormal findings would represent conditions outside the scope of scientifically validated chiropractic treatment, such tests would be more appropriately administered and interpreted by medical doctors than by chiropractors. In fact, they are a standard part of good medical practice. They do not, however, provide a legitimate basis for prescribing supplements.

"Nutrient Deficiency" Questionnaires

Many questionnaires have been devised to help persuade people they need supplements. Some have been distributed by companies that market supplements through chiropractors. Others have been devised and distributed by independent entrepreneurs. Some contain only a brief list of questions, while others contain more than a hundred. Some questionnaires are related to ideas that extra nutrients are needed to cope with factors in people's lifestyle or environment. Others include symptoms supposedly related to "nutrient deficiencies." The more elaborate questionnaires are scored by a computer operated by the chiropractor or the company marketing the test. The computers are programmed to recommend supplements for everyone, usually a long list of them. Barrett and Herbert have summed up the situation this way:

> Nutrition professionals may use a questionnaire as part of an evaluation for dietary counseling. But no questionnaire can provide a legitimate basis for prescribing dietary supplements. Questionnaires covering symptoms, illnesses, health habits, and other lifestyle factors can be a valuable part of a comprehensive medical evaluation. However, symptom-based questionnaires used for the purpose of providing supplement recommendations are invariably bogus. [25]

Overview

How accurately does the information in this chapter reflect what chiropractors are doing about nutrition? Are many chiropractors involved in the delivery of appropriate nutritional advice to their patients? Are things likely to improve in the future?

In 1992, Ira Milner, R.D., examined catalogs from chiropractic colleges, wrote for detailed information about their nutrition courses, and made additional inquiries by phone. Each of the seventeen schools offered at least one course. Thirteen taught basic nutrition, and fourteen had at least one course in clinical nutrition. Some schools did not reply to Milner's inquiry, and some refused to provide information. Of those that did provide information, some used standard nutrition textbooks, some used nonstandard books, and some used a mixture of the two.

Dr. Barrett has been monitoring the chiropractic marketplace for more than twenty-five years and probably has the largest collection of chiropractic books, journals, and other literature outside chiropractic hands. While editing this book, he provided me with the following observations:

- The American Chiropractic Association and the International Chiropractors Association do not appear to be encouraging their members to do appropriate nutrition counseling. Neither group has endorsed water fluoridation. (The ACA has ducked the issue, while the ICA is opposed.) The "journal" of the ACA Council on Nutrition promotes many quack ideas and carries many ads from supplement companies that market questionable products. Several years ago, the ACA condemned cytotoxic testing (a phony test for food allergies), but this action was taken after government agencies had virtually driven the test from the marketplace. The council has failed to criticize hair analysis or any other quack practice widely used by chiropractors. It has also cosponsored seminars on "The Subluxation Complex: Neurological and Nutritional Considerations," which provide information on how diet and nutritional supplementation can inhibit the production of "the chemical irritants that perpetuate subluxations." The ACA's 508-page *Basic Principles of Chiropractic* maintains that testing the pH of saliva can determine whether the sympathetic or parasympathetic nervous system is overactive and whether "phosphorus deficiency" is present. The book also contains nonsensical charts on the "projected effects of subluxations" on the metabolism of carbohydrates, fat, protein, and water [212].

- If properly informed, chiropractors could legitimately advise patients on: (a) general dietary guidelines, (b) how to consume sufficient calcium to help prevent osteoporosis, (c) how to consume adequate amounts of fiber to help prevent certain types of cancer, (d) appropriate weight-control measures, and (e) the importance of adequate fluoride intake for preventing tooth decay. Chiropractors might also become able to check blood cholesterol levels and advise patients accordingly. The amount of information on these subjects reaching chiropractors through their journals is very small.

• During the past few years, several prominent medical textbook publishers have issued books written or edited by chiropractic educators and intended for use by students and practitioners. The scope and quality of these books vary enormously. Only one book I have seen provides the basic facts on each of the above topics and offers practical advice for helping patients [117]. Another covers most of this in superb detail, but goes astray on diet and hyperactivity [210]. Another includes a page on laboratory evaluation of nutritional status but contains only useless and misleading generalities [96]. A large clinical text on "chiropractic family practice" contains less than a page on "nutrition." It discusses "innate intelligence and nutritional therapy" and advises that "for the vast majority of patients, nutritional intervention is of crucial importance" in correcting subluxations [243]. A companion "patient resource manual" provides well-designed diet assessment sheets but reprints a health-food newsletter's unfounded advice on "enhancing the immune system" with supplements [142]. Yet another large text lists recommendations from the *Surgeon General's Report on Nutrition* plus guidance on how to increase fiber and lower the fat and cholesterol content of one's diet. But it also states that nutritional supplementation is "integral to the management of visceral [nonmusculoskeletal] and other disorders ... to support the healing of tissues affected by the vertebral subluxation complex" [194]. A clinical handbook makes inappropriate supplement recommendations throughout its nutrition chapter [257]. And a nutrition handbook provides a confusing mixture of facts, speculations, and unsubstantiated advice, including protocols for some conditions that chiropractors should not be treating [85].

• *Dynamic Chiropractic* maintains a computerized list of scheduled seminars. During 1994, judging from their titles, no more than seven out of about two thousand were on scientific aspects of nutrition.

• A 1995 pamphlet from the Foundation for Chiropractic Education and Research advises: "If you do not feel you are getting the most of your diet, or if you feel your digestive process is generally faulty, consider consulting your Doctor of Chiropractic who can determine if your digestive concerns involve interference in the nervous system" [64]. The likelihood that a digestive problem is due to "interference in the nervous system" correctable by a chiropractor is zero. The pamphlet also contends that "many times, therapeutic supplements are prescribed by Doctors of Chiropractic to enhance the healing of injuries or illness." The fact that these prescriptions are almost always inappropriate is not mentioned.

• At the July 1995 Chiropractic Centennial Celebration held in Washington, D.C., eighteen of the 166 exhibitors hawked dubious supplement and/or herbal products and two demonstrated and marketed equipment for live cell analysis.

Jennifer R. Jamison, M.B., B.Ch., M.Ed., M.Sc., a physician who heads the department of diagnostic science at an Australian school of chiropractic and osteopathy, has stated: "Nutritional supplementation cannot be regarded as an inherently drugless form of clinical intervention. When prescribed in megadoses, nutrients should be construed as pharmaceuticals" [116]. To the inevitable response that megadoses of nutrients should not be considered drugs because they are "natural" and harmless, she points out that the drug hydrocortisone is also natural, yet able to produce serious side effects. And so can high doses of nutrients.

Excessive amounts of vitamin A, for example, can damage the liver, vitamin C can cause diarrhea, and vitamin B_6 can cause nerve toxicity. The number of reported cases may not be large, but when supplements are prescribed for senseless reasons—as many chiropractors are prone to do— the chance of their helping is zero. Regardless of how little risk may be involved, the odds don't justify their use for incorrect reasons. Nor do ethical considerations.

The Bottom Line

"Nutritional therapy" is chiropractic's "alternative" to the drugs prescribed by the medical profession. The nutrition-related diagnostic and treatment systems used by chiropractors are foolish and exploit patients. I don't know whether "chiropractic nutrition" is motivated more by delusion or by greed. Regardless, sound nutrition advice, when needed, can easily be obtained elsewhere.

9

Should Chiropractors Treat Children?

The percentage of chiropractors who treat children and the manner in which they do so has not been systematically studied. But there are good reasons to be suspicious. Chiropractic schooling in pediatric diagnosis is scanty (see Chapter 4). Few childhood ailments are legitimately within chiropractic's scope. Many chiropractors exaggerate what they can do. And, as noted in Chapter 14, many advise against immunization and other proven public health measures.

Dubious Claims

Many chiropractors and their organizations recommend chiropractic care throughout childhood. The sales pitches used are similar to those for adults.

• During the 1970s, the American Chiropractic Association (ACA) said that, "Everyone needs a periodic spinal examination . . . especially kids!" During the mid-1980s, an ACA ad asked why children should have chiropractic manipulation and answered: "Because growth and development can be affected by minor bumps, jars and falls."

• A 1976 chiropractic text by W.W. Stierwalt, D.C., assistant professor of technique at Palmer College, claimed that crankiness in an apparently healthy infant may signify a "subluxation" that, if removed, will give the infant a "new outlook on Life" [239].

• "Your Children Deserve Chiropractic Care," a 1976 pamphlet from the Sherman College of Straight Chiropractic, asserted that the body's "internal balance can only be restored when the internal interference to the nervous system is removed.... The result of internal balance will allow *your children to be the ancestors of a better humanity,* so that subsequent generations will be consciously superior physically, mentally, and socially."

• A 1977 Parker Research Foundation pamphlet titled "Chiropractic helps children develop into healthy adults" contended that "7 out of 10 children show definite spinal distortions" and that colic, bed-wetting, hyperactivity, skin rashes, asthma, and upset stomach can be caused by

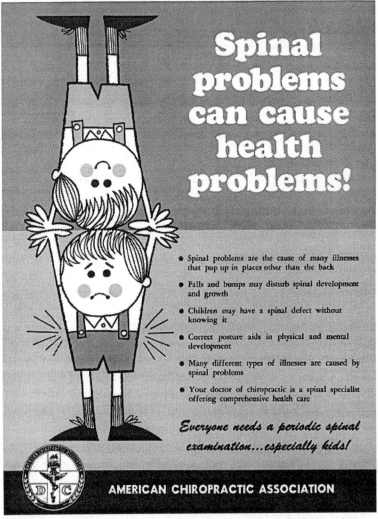

Poster distributed by the American Chiropractic Association since the mid-1970s. Every statement in the ad is either false or misleading.

"nerve interference" that chiropractors can correct. Another Parker pamphlet, "Your Children May Inherit Your Spinal Weakness," contends: "A regular spinal examination at least once a year during your child's growing years is one of the best physical health insurance procedures you can obtain for him."

• A recent pamphlet from Singer and Associates claims: "Many childhood ailments that used to be passed off as 'phases' a child goes through . . . are now being traced to spinal misalignments."

• Ted Koren, D.C., who publishes a large line of flyers for chiropractic offices, contends that "a spinal check-up for your child could be one of the most important check-ups in his or her life." His 1987 "Children and Chiropractic" brochure lists thirty-three "common disorders in children which are remarkably helped by chiropractic." The list includes fever, high blood pressure, sore throat, bronchitis, poor concentration, loss of hearing, eye problems, skin disorders, croup, ear infections, nervousness, and cough.

• Louis Sportelli, D.C., a former chairman of the ACA's board of governors, has written and published *Introduction to Chiropractic*, a booklet which asserts that "regular spinal adjustments are a part of your body's defense against illness." The ninth edition, which was distributed by the ACA, states:

> The strains to which children are subject can easily be a contributing factor in creating spinal malfunctions (subluxations) and/or nerve irritation. . . . Clinical evidence suggests that common disorders of childhood such as colds, constipation, asthma, and other conditions can be helped through spinal manipulations (adjustments) if they are the result of neurological irritations caused by spinal imbalances. . . .
>
> If parents were as concerned about having their children's spines checked for minor derangements (subluxations) as they are about having their children's teeth checked for cavities, they would be helping their youngsters attain a healthier state of well-being. Proper spinal care is essential to your child's health.

No mention is made of the obvious fact that most children do quite well without spinal manipulation.

• In a 1990 policy statement, the International Chiropractors Association (ICA) advised "the earliest possible evaluation, detection and correction of chiropractic lesions (subluxations) in children, especially infants, to maximize the potential for normal growth and development." The ICA even holds an annual National Conference on Chiropractic & Pediatrics and has a three-hundred-hour Diplomate in Chiropractic Pediatrics program to provide "quality education in pediatrics."

• In 1992, the ICA released a videotape called "Chiropractic and Your Child: A Partnership for the Future." Intended for viewing in chiropractic offices, it asserts that: (1) pediatricians typically diagnose and treat disease with little emphasis on prevention; (2) subluxations arise from "falls, blows, birth trauma, and normal daily living"; (3) standard medical treatment for middle-ear infections is ineffective and can produce significant side effects; (4) middle-ear infections are caused by subluxations of the bones of the neck and head; (5) chiropractic treatment can help prevent such infections; and (6) chiropractors are primary-care physicians who are able to determine what is wrong and what type of care is needed. These views are not merely unsubstantiated; the statement that prevention is not emphasized by pediatricians—who, of course, vigorously support immunization—is a bare-faced lie.

• Recently, the ICA published a brochure titled, "When should you take your child to a Chiropractor? A Parent's Guide to Chiropractic." The brochure describes four circumstances: (1) When you want your child to have all the benefits of a conservative, drugless approach to health care, (2) When you want to give your child a head start in good health, (3) When your child takes a fall, and (4) When your child takes part in athletic activities.

• "Babies & Children," a 1993 flyer from Activator Methods, Inc., contends that for painful and difficult ear infections, chiropractic evaluation may be "most helpful when evaluating stubborn repeat infections or when conservative treatment is preferable to medication or surgery."

"Where Is the Subluxation?" is about a little girl who was told she had a subluxation and searched in vain under her bed and in her toybox to find it. She finally learned its location when the chiropractor said it was a bone in her neck that was "not lined up with the other ones." The chiropractor explained: "Subluxations make your body sick. Each time I push on your back, the bones are adjusted closer to their normal position. This opens up the pathways, so that your brain may talk properly with your body. As your subluxations are corrected, you become healthier." The booklet was written by Jennifer Peet, D.C., and published in 1992.

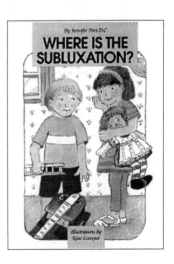

• Palmer and Jennifer Peet practice in South Burlington, Vermont, and operate The Baby Adjusters, a chiropractic supply firm. The Peets also teach in the certification program in chiropractic pediatrics cosponsored by Life College and the International Chiropractic Pediatrics Association. During recent interviews, the Peets stated that they adjusted the spines of two to three hundred patients a day, mostly children and some infants, and that "chiropractors are seeing that if you start young with a child you have a better chance to improve their well-being." Their pamphlet, "Should your children have a chiropractic check-up?" states that newborns should be checked for subluxations "within hours after birth." Palmer's foreword to the second edition of Jennifer's three-hundred-page *Chiropractic Pediatric & Prenatal Reference Manual* states:

> In your practice right now, you probably have children that are developing colon cancer, that will manifest in 50 years if you don't adjust them now. . . . Now is the time to tell your patients that subluxations are slowly killing their children. The time is now to start adjusting children from birth. . . . One should never underestimate the power of the chiropractic adjustment. Use the information within this book to give your best adjustments to infants and children. Then all the power in heaven will break loose within them and miraculous healings will occur on a daily basis. [187]

The book also claims that "the dangers of vaccinations to the young child are profound" and that "in some cases, the vaccine acts nonspecifically [sic] to increase a child's preexisting chronic disease tendency." The book concludes: "Every time a child receives a chiropractic adjustment it should be given as if their very life depends on it, because it does."

• The Peets appear to recommend that every child be examined repeatedly with x-rays. Jennifer's reference manual states:

> Subluxations can be life-threatening. Chiropractors should not hesitate to take whatever radiographs are necessary to completely analyze the subluxation complex the child presents. Without radiographs, the effects of spinal adjustments cannot be completely evaluated. [186:115]

• Peter Pan Potential, cofounded by Claudia Anrig Howe, D.C., offers seminars for "a comprehensive program covering all aspects of pediatric chiropractic." In a recent article, she advised: "Many of our colleagues cry out for new ideas to survive in practice, when right under their noses lies the answer. Go to the children" [112]. She suggests that an interest in treating children be communicated by asking prospective patients who phone for an appointment whether it is for themself or a child. She also suggests telling adults that "spinal degeneration" is related to "the Vertebral Subluxation Complex undetected and uncorrected as a child."

• Howe has also contributed a chapter to the *Textbook of Clinical Chiropractic,* a book published by Williams & Wilkins, a prominent medical publisher [111]. Her chapter emphasizes the detection and adjustment of "subluxations" and the "chiropractic evaluation" of common pediatric disorders. The conditions discussed are colds and other upper respiratory infections, colic, digestive disorders, bedwetting, febrile convulsions, abnormal rotations of the foot, growing pains, headache, jaundice, otitis media (inflammation of the middle ear), scoliosis, tonsillitis, torticollis (wry neck), attention deficit disorder ("hyperactivity"), cerebral palsy, Down's syndrome, and epilepsy. For most, Howe includes a superficial description of signs and symptoms plus tips for locating subluxations. She ignores the fact that some of these conditions should have urgent medical attention. She contends:

> Subluxation of the spinal column and its reduction with an adjustment is considered of benefit to the patient, regardless of the presenting symptoms, if any. This approach is not to be interpreted as the remedy of all disease, but rather, a way to enhance the individual's potential for normal function.

• Another large Williams & Wilkins textbook contains a twenty-one-page chapter on pediatric disorders written by Randy L. Swenson, D.C., a professor of chiropractic and academic dean at the National College of Chiropractic [244]. After reviewing its contents, Dr. Stephen Barrett provided me with the following comments:

> Swenson writes as though it is appropriate for chiropractors to assume the management of many types of illnesses and refer to "other health care practitioners" when extra help is needed. He recommends manipulation for conjunctivitis, sinusitis, sore throats, tonsillitis, otitis media, croup, asthma, colic, constipation, diarrhea, epilepsy, scoliosis, synovitis (joint inflammation), and the normal "spitting up" of food by infants. For tonsillitis, he also recommends massaging the tonsils and painting them with an iodine solution "to kill surface bacteria." For croup, he recommends acupuncture. Although he indicates that some of these conditions require medical care, he gives little advice on how to determine which children need it. For example, he fails to indicate that antibiotic therapy should be administered in bacterial infections of the ear or eye, including the case of a child pictured in the book with one eye swollen shut by a severe infection!

For epilepsy, the book states, "chiropractic care should also be offered as an opportunity to maintain freedom from medications, such as phenobarbital, which are deleterious to the mental development of children if used for too long a time period."

The passage on immunization states that "immunization programs continue on the premise of prevention," but "it cannot be said that the . . . program has been proven successful . . . and the complication rates for the vaccines continues to claim the lives of children via disability and/or death." The passage also contends that "the very long-term effects . . . may not be known until well into the next century."

Swenson states correctly that croup due to *Hemophilus influenzae* type B is a medical emergency and can be diagnosed by noting that the child's epiglottis is a cherry-red color and may be easy to see. But he fails to warn that if an infected child is in acute respiratory distress, examining the epiglottis can cause death. Nor does Swenson include *Hemophilus influenzae* type B in his discussion of "immunizable contagious diseases," even though an effective vaccine was approved by the FDA in 1985, more than five years before the book was published.

Quite frankly, I am shocked by the poor quality of this chapter and the fact that a major medical publisher would print it.

Undercover Investigations

Three investigations have been conducted in which a child was taken to chiropractors while an adult recorded what happened. In 1973, four-year-old Cindy Roseberry visited five chiropractors in Eastern Pennsylvania for a checkup. Cindy was apparently healthy and had experienced no serious illnesses. Before the investigation began, she was examined by a local pediatrician, who found no abnormalities. The first chiropractor examined Cindy for about a minute by running a "Nervo-Scope" up and down her spine. He reported "pinched nerves to her stomach and gallbladder" and said that her shoulder blades were "out of place." He advised having an x-ray examination, which he said involved less radiation than three hours in the sun. He also said that his own little girl underwent weekly adjustments. The second chiropractor showed a movie which stated that "chiropractic can also be effective in combating most childhood diseases." He said that Cindy's pelvis was "twisted" and advised that she have "adjustments, vitamins, and a check every four months." The third chiropractor said that one hip was "elevated" and that spinal misalignments could cause Cindy to develop "headaches, nervousness, equilibrium or digestive problems" in the future. He advised getting an x-ray to see whether some "weakness" was minor or serious. He also said that chiropractic analysis shows if there was a vitamin lacking and that "there are over twenty-six different vitamins." (There are actually thirteen.) The fourth chiropractor predicted "bad periods and rough childbirth" if Cindy's "shorter left leg" were not treated. He also found "tension in the neck." He said he adjusted his own family once a week and recommended weekly checkups and adjustments for everyone else. The fifth chiropractor not only found hip and neck misalignments, but also "adjusted" them without asking permission. The adjustments were so painful that the investigation was terminated [18].

In February 1994, ABC's "20/20" reported on visits to seventeen chiropractors who had made it known through advertising or other means that they treated children. In one segment, an infant named Blake was taken by his mother to nine chiropractors in the New York metropolitan area, accompanied by a "friend" who was carrying a hidden camera. Blake had had recurring ear infections, a problem that a pediatrician said could be managed with antibiotics and would eventually be outgrown. Every one of the chiropractors found a problem, and all nine said they could help and recommended care ranging from several weeks to a lifetime. The first found "a misalignment between the second and third bones in his neck." The second said it was "on the right side of his neck between the first and second bones." The third, using muscle-testing, found "weakness in the adrenal glands." The fourth said there was a subluxation because one of Blake's legs was shorter than the other. The fifth claimed he could diagnose the boy's problem by pulling on *his mother's* arm while she touched the boy on the shoulder. The sixth chiropractor did a similar test by pulling on the mother's legs while Blake lay on top of her back. After diagnosing "jamming of the occiput (the back bone of the skull)," the chiropractor said he corrected it by "lifting" Blake's occiput with his thumbs. He also said: (a) Blake needed work on his immune system, (b) learning disorder might be a problem, (c) both mother and son had "eyes that don't team too well," and (d) the cameraman, whom the chiropractor incorrectly assumed was the boy's father, had the same eye problem.

The same program also reported on visits to eight Wisconsin chiropractors by a five-year-old boy with chronic ear infections so severe that medical doctors wanted to insert tubes in his ears to drain them. All eight chiropractors found problems, but not usually the same ones. One diagnosed a pinched nerve in the boy's neck. Another said his left leg was shorter than his right. Another said his right leg was shorter than his left. Another diagnosed zinc deficiency. Another chiropractor blamed the boy's ear problems on "food sensitivities" and advised avoiding corn, cow's milk, and white flour. Another chiropractor gave similar dietary advice but said that the main diagnosis was a "subluxation" in the top vertebra. Another said the boy didn't have an ear problem but had scoliosis—a diagnosis disputed by a pediatrician and a radiologist who reviewed this chiropractor's findings.

These investigations illustrate three things. First, a large percentage of chiropractors who treat children use bizarre diagnostic methods and diagnose nonexistent problems. Second, when confronted with a child who has a real illness, a large percentage will recommend incorrect treatment. Third, chiropractic is not a science; for if it were, the diagnoses would not have varied wildly.

Treatment of Ear Infections

Many chiropractors claim they can treat ear infections. In March 1993, the *Wall Street Journal* reported that a five-year-old boy and his four-year-old sister had developed mastoiditis, a condition due to a middle-ear infection so advanced that it invades the skull [233]. Thanks to antibiotics, mastoiditis is rarely seen in this country. But these children had been diagnosed and their care managed by a chiropractor who treated them with spinal manipulation. The children should have been referred to a medical doctor for antibiotic therapy. Instead, both became seriously ill, and the girl lost her hearing in one ear. The report gave chiropractic such a black eye that the ACA placed a full-page ad in the *Wall Street Journal* stating that "any doctor of chiropractic who would seek to substitute spinal manipulation for antibiotic therapy in the treatment of bacterial infections . . . is acting counter to accepted clinical practices."

A few months later, Paul Brown, M.D., an internist who practices in Minnesota, surveyed chiropractic offices in the Minneapolis-St. Paul area. He began with the first chiropractic listing in the Yellow Pages and phoned until he had one hundred complete responses. Posing as the parent of a four-year-old child with ear problems, he asked whether the chiropractor treated children and ear infections. All but one replied that the chiropractor treated children, and eighty said that the chiropractor treated ear infections. Some chiropractors said that ear problems occur because the first cervical vertebra often is out of place and thereby affects nerves and blood vessels. Others claimed that dietary problems such as consumption of cow's milk leads to excessive mucus production, which also contributes to the problem [19]. This claim has no scientific substantiation.

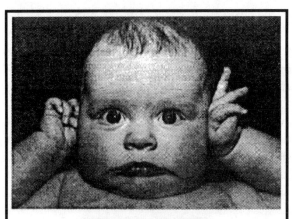
This ad appeared in April 1993 in a newspaper in Pennsylvania. The *JAMA* article mentioned in item #2 was not about acute or painful ear infections. It concerned serous otitis, a *painless* collection of fluid in the middle ear.

I believe it is risky to rely on chiropractic treatment for ear problems. Acute middle-ear infections should be treated promptly with antibiotics. Recurrent infections and other chronic ear problems require sophisticated medical attention. Chiropractors have no business monkeying with them.

The Foundation for Chiropractic Education and Research suggests otherwise in "Chiropractic and the Pediatric Patient," a 1993 videotape it distributes to chiropractors. In one segment, a chiropractor who taught pediatrics at a chiropractic college described how she treated chronic ear infections with spinal and cranial adjustments, homeopathic remedies ("to help build the immune system that has been altered with the use of antibiotics"), and dietary changes such as elimination of dairy products. Acknowledging that chiropractors are not pediatricians, she said parents should be encouraged to "keep a pediatrician on staff that is always ready to take over when needed."

Seductive Marketing Tactics

In 1992, a reporter who attended an "aJust Kids" seminar sponsored by the American Academy of Chiropractic Pediatrics obtained materials that included twenty-one "pediatric practice ideas." The ideas, written in a child's "voice," included:

- Us kids need chiropractic care as much as anyone else. Why aren't there more children in your chiropractic office? The most obvious reason is that you have not been able to educate mom, dad, family and other adults.

- Adjust us on a pediatric adjusting table in the waiting room and watch how easy it will be to educate everybody.

Straight Status, Inc., of New Castle, Indiana, calls its products "the fun alternative for patient-pleasing practice promotion." It offers a large line of office apparel, sportswear, greeting cards, stickers, bookmarks, and other novelty items. After noting that "kids are the future of chiropractic," its catalog states: "Introducing the benefits of chiropractic care to children at an early age promotes a lifetime of good health care and builds patient loyalty that will last a long time.... Our colorful designs will attract the attention of all young patients .... When displayed in the office, parents will inquire about 'Kids and Chiropractic.'"

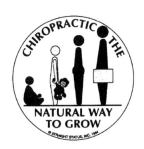

- Take 2 polaroid pictures of the Doctor and me on a pediatric adjusting table. Put a copy on the kids wall and give the other to me to take home (I will share it with everyone I know).

- Have a "Draw the Spine" or "Color the Spine" . . . contest. Award prizes, we love prizes, lots of prizes.

- Have a graduation ceremony (DIPLOMA) when we graduate to a larger table.

- Love us, hug us, and play with us kids. Do this on our level, we have no understanding of your level.

- Give us gift certificates for referring patients.

- Talk about child abuse and neglect. Worse [sic] child neglect in the world is not getting our subluxations adjusted.

- Give us a little luv and you will get back much more.

Considerable Risk, Little or No Benefit

The evidence that "chiropractic pediatrics" can be dangerous is substantial. For example, a four-month-old boy with torticollis was paralyzed immediately after a chiropractic neck manipulation [217]. The chiropractor had missed a large tumor near the child's spinal cord and is believed to have ruptured it with an adjustment. Doctors in Marshfield, Wisconsin, reported on more than a dozen children who were misdiagnosed and inappropriately treated while serious conditions continued or worsened. Four of the children had cancer [172]. The undercover investigations described earlier in this chapter indicate that many chiropractors are making absurd diagnoses in both sick and healthy children and some are exposing children to large doses of unnecessary x-radiation. In addition, there are the potentially deadly risks created by chiropractors who disparage responsible immunization, antibiotic therapy, and medical care in general.

There are also psychologic and financial dangers. What do you suppose takes place in the minds of children who have monthly or even weekly treatment for the "subluxations," "leg-length inequalities," "energy imbalances," or the other delusional concepts described in Chapters 7 and 8 of this book? What do you suppose is the impact of being forced to take laxatives, herbs, and/or dietary supplement concoctions, as described in

Appendix A? What do you think happens when a chiropractor plays with, praises, and hugs children for being "good patients" and uses them for marketing purposes? And what about the thousands of dollars that this "treatment" costs?

Numerous informed voices have been raised in opposition to "chiropractic pediatrics." Reformist Peter Modde, D.C., has warned that "the treatment of diseases of infants and children is a complex undertaking that for the untrained holds many surprises and dangers. It is . . . improper care for a chiropractor to style himself a chiropractic pediatrician, professing a medical ability to detect and treat childhood infections and other specific disorders of the young" [164:222].

Jeff Young, D.O., an osteopathic pediatrician who uses manipulative therapy, told a *Consumer Reports* editor that preventive maintenance adjustments on children have "absolutely no medical data to support them," and that "there is no research to justify its use in the treatment of epilepsy, asthma, bedwetting, or learning disabilities, some of the many childhood problems for which chiropractic claims are made" [47].

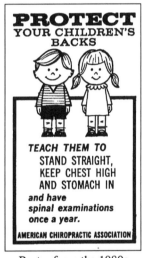

Poster from the 1980s

Many chiropractors conduct "screenings" in which they evaluate children's posture and look for cases of scoliosis (abnormal sideward curvature of the spine). *Consumer Reports* took a slap at this practice with the comment: "Correct Posture Month aside, manipulation won't correct a habit such as slouched shoulders or affect the progression of scoliosis" [47]. Most cases of spinal curvature do not progress, and for those that do, bracing or surgery are the only proven treatments.

Murray Katz, M.D.C.M., who directs the largest pediatric clinic in Canada and advocates manipulative therapy for musculoskeletal problems in adults, states flatly that manipulation is inappropriate for infants and children and that much of the chiropractic treatment of children is pretense. In 1992, three researchers from the neuroscience department of the University of Illinois College of Medicine concluded that, "Potential complications and unknown benefits indicate that spinal manipulative therapy should not be used in the pediatric population" [199]. Modde seems to sum up the situation best:

Chiropractic pediatrics is a dangerous, false profession. There is no scientific medical proof that chiropractic has any efficacy against childhood diseases. Although chiropractors report positive results in treating children for many conditions, one must always wonder whether the diagnosis was accurate and whether the chiropractic treatment had anything to do with the reported recovery. Chiropractors receive some pediatric training, but there is a severe danger of their not recognizing problems that need medical attention. [164:203]

10

Insurance Abuses

Chiropractic services are covered to some extent under Medicare, Medicaid, workers' compensation, and most commercial health insurance plans. This represents political recognition but has nothing whatever to do with scientific legitimacy. Insurance companies are generally willing to cover treatments that the scientific community recognizes as effective. Insurance plans usually cover services considered "reasonable and necessary." As this book illustrates, many chiropractic services fail to meet these criteria. Medicare coverage was gained in 1973 through a massive lobbying campaign. Most coverage in commercial insurance and other nongovernmental plans was gained through passage of "insurance equality" laws that force insurers to cover chiropractic whether they want to do so or not. Most prefer not to do so, for reasons discussed in this chapter.

In some states, health maintenance organizations (HMOs) have also been forced to include chiropractors. However, very few of them do so without payment limits and other restrictions such as requiring medical referral. The largest HMO, Kaiser Permanente, does not cover chiropractic care [140].

The Medicare Paradox

Richard D. Lyons, a staff writer for the *New York Times*, has poignantly described the events leading to chiropractic inclusion under Medicare:

127

After seven years of ceaseless lobbying, chiropractors have finally succeeded in getting themselves included in the multibillion-dollar Medicare program through a series of events that offers a view of the workings of Washington in microcosm.

The cast of characters involves the small but determined band of chiropractors, their patients, lobbyists for and against their cause, Senators and Representatives, federal officials, campaign contributions, and tens of thousands if not millions of pieces of mail. . . .

Staff aids at the two congressional committees that dealt with the chiropractic legislation . . . expressed astonishment over the sacks of mail that never seemed to diminish, in contrast to other issues that peaked and were then forgotten. [154]

The law, which was enacted in 1972 and took effect in 1973, limited coverage to manual manipulation of the spine for "subluxations demonstrated by x-rays to exist." Since the chiropractic "subluxation" is visible only to chiropractors, this could have posed a serious problem. But federal officials concluded that Congress intended Medicare to pay for *something* and accepted a loosely worded chiropractic "definition" of subluxations for which payment could be made: "an incomplete dislocation, off-centering, fixation or abnormal spacing of the vertebrae . . . demonstrable . . . to individuals trained in the reading of x-rays." A *New York Times* editorial called the enactment of Medicare coverage "the most shocking victory for special-interest lobbyists" and added that "the scientific basis of the chiropractic cult is highly dubious" [103].

In 1986, a report from the U.S. Department of Health and Human Services' Office of the Inspector General (OIG) revealed that Medicare payments to chiropractors had expanded at the rate of 18.7 percent per year between 1975 and 1984 and that chiropractic manipulation had been the ninth most frequently billed procedure under Medicare during 1983. The report noted:

The Medicare Carriers Manual . . . presents a system for classifying subluxations . . . and a system for relating various symptoms to a particular area of the spine. The manual also lists examples of conditions for which manual manipulation of the spine is *not* an appropriate treatment. Some critics have suggested that this system has provided a blueprint for chiropractors to work backward to identify the appropriate location of a subluxation for billing purposes, as opposed to treating and billing for a subluxation which has been identified on an x-ray. [167]

Table 6-1. Status of Medicare Claims, 1981–1985

Fiscal Year	Claims Received	Number Denied or Partially Denied	Total Amount of Claims	Total Amount Disallowed	Amount Paid
1981	1,592,278	716,775 (45.0%)	$105,999,620	$43,555,118 (41.1%)	$62,444,502
1982	1,890,941	807,622 (42.7%)	128,798,353	55,186,021 (42.8%)	73,612,332
1983	2,162,077	951,571 (44.0%)	156,051,606	72,187,272 (46.3%)	83,863,334
1984	2,355,055	1,040,277 (44.2%)	171,427,024	78,839,266 (46.0%)	92,587,758
1985	2,798,290	1,233,357 (44.1%)	197,287,803	97,391,115 (49.4%)	99,896,688

Indeed, when OIG investigators surveyed 145 chiropractors by telephone, 84 percent said that some subluxations do not show on x-rays, but nearly half responded that when billing Medicare, they "could always find something" (by x-ray or physical examination) to justify the diagnosis, or actually tailored the diagnosis to obtain reimbursement. The OIG concluded that "the x-ray requirement is not currently well enforced, may be unenforceable and is highly conducive to abuse" [167].

By requiring x-ray examinations to document something that does not exist, our government is promoting diagnostically worthless irradiation of millions of innocent patients. X-rays can cause cancer, and there is no totally safe minimum dose. The public loses both healthwise, and in paying for the treatment of chiropractic illusions. The table above shows how Medicare payments grew between 1981 and 1985, as well as the percentage of claims that were denied or partially denied. The total payout has continued to outpace inflation, reaching $181 million in 1990.

Other Insurance Plans

Sociologist Walter Wardwell, Ph.D., a strong chiropractic sympathizer, believes that insurance companies should benefit from covering chiropractic services:

> If it is less costly to reimburse chiropractors than M.D.s, insurance companies should not be reluctant to reimburse them for almost anything they do. Even if they believe that chiropractic benefits are

due only to a placebo effect, they should find it advantageous to reimburse. (While it may not be a flattering comparison, some insurance companies have even reimbursed Christian Science practitioners for their services, presumably because it saved them money.) [255:264]

Most insurers, however, do not believe that chiropractic coverage is cost-effective—and most are also concerned about overbilling.

The most extreme and well documented example of overbilling occurred during the early 1960s. The National Association of Letter Carriers included chiropractic in its health benefits plan in 1960 but dropped it five years later [62]. Charles K. Holmes, M.D., the plan's medical director, described the experience as "a nightmare of catastrophic proportions." In a report sent to Dr. Stephen Barrett in 1970, he stated:

While supposed to limit chiropractic to conditions of the spine, [they] were treating every disease known to man. Their diagnoses included measles, mumps, cardiac disease, duodenal ulcer . . . cancer of the prostate, mental disease, nocturnal enuresis, gynecological conditions . . . and a host of others, all supposed to result from claimed subluxations of a vertebra. [90]

Holmes's report included copies of bills for the following:

- 10 treatments, an x-ray exam, and two bottles of B-complex vitamins for angina pectoris (over a five-week period)
- 18 treatments and an x-ray exam for mumps (ten weeks)
- 29 treatments and an x-ray exam for bedwetting (nine months)
- 49 treatments for "craniospinal nerve pressure" (one year)
- 66 treatments, including fifteen for "gallbladder," twenty-seven for "respiratory," seven for "acute traumatic cervical myofascitis," and seventeen for "gallbladder, cervical strain" (one year)
- 81 treatments for duodenal ulcer (eleven months).

Although chiropractic billing practices have improved considerably since the 1960s, inappropriate billing is by no means rare. In 1985, the sixteen-person individual health insurance committee of the International Claim Association held a workshop on "gimmicks, gadgets and fads" that were causing problems for their companies. The committee's report stated:

There are hundreds of theories without scientific basis for which governments and insurance companies pay millions of dollars every year. The companies are often torn between insurance departments, health agencies and . . . legislatures demanding "cost control" on one hand and on the other hand facing the possibility of being penalized millions of dollars in punitive damages if they attempt to practice any cost control.

Most of the problem areas involved chiropractors. The report criticized thermography, contour analysis, applied kinesiology, skin-temperature gadgets used to diagnose "subluxations," hair analysis, nutritional counseling, and hand-held "adjusting" devices such as the Activator. (Each of these is described in Chapters 7 or 8 and the glossary of this book.) The report also stated:

> Especially in the area of chiropractic claims, gimmick billing has reached the level of fine art. Practice-building courses coach chiropractors on what to say to patients – and to insurance companies.
>
> Seven claims received from the same chiropractor indicate what "practice building" can do. For practical purposes the diagnoses were identical:
> a. All were diagnosed as having "paresthesia."
> b. Four had "occipital cephalalgia."
> c. Four had "cervical radiculitis."
> d. Two had "lumbalgia" (an illness you won't find in your medical dictionary).
> e. One had occipital neuritis, one sciatic neuritis.
> f. Four claims had two identical x-ray exams. . . .
> g. Each had three diagnoses.
> h. All had completed "no out of pocket" assignments.
> i. The lowest bill was $820.00, the highest $2,510.00, average $1,556.00.
> j. Of the total $10,895 charges, only $2,920 could be substantiated by the doctor's records.
>
> Actually an offshoot of billing gimmicks, the ultimate billing program is the "no out of pocket" system. The practitioner simply agrees to accept whatever the insurance pays so the patient has no out-of-pocket expenses no matter how much treatment he receives. . . . State legislatures are slowly outlawing the practice.

In 1986, at a meeting of the National Health Care Anti-Fraud Association, Dr. Barrett asked a large audience of senior claims examiners about their experiences with chiropractic claims. When he asked whether any of them were *not* having trouble, not a single hand went up [23].

The most frequent problem appears to be unnecessary treatment. During the early 1980s, for example, researchers who conducted a large survey of back-pain sufferers concluded that "the high cost of chiropractic care . . . bothered survey participants most—not the cost per visit but the long-range nature of the treatment" [136:61]. In 1990, a chiropractor who met with claims adjusters from the California State Automobile Association reported:

> [The adjusters] believe that once patients are permanent and stable we should discharge them. Yet they have seen bills from many chiropractors who have treated patients for years. . . . Many chiropractors have continued treatment long after patients are asymptomatic. The adjusters' complaints were substantiated by stacks of bills they showed me from chiropractors who were providing treatment without any rationale or any regular report of progress. I saw bills for $70 or $80 per visit, for two or three visits per week, for as long as two or three years. [248]

During a 1995 interview, the head of fraud detection for a large Blue Cross/Blue Shield plan told Barrett:

> We rarely see claims where the patient goes once or twice. Most seem to keep going until they reach the limits of their coverage. Then they are told they are cured. We also get claims for the treatment of "subluxations" in cases where we know the patient's problem is cancer or another disease that is nowhere within the scope of chiropractic. The claim forms don't show it, but we know that some of these patients are being told that fixing their "subluxation" can make them better.

Overbilling has even been addressed by Sid E. Williams, D.C., president of Life College, a leading proponent of lifetime chiropractic care for "preventive maintenance" (see Chapter 6). In a 1992 plea for a "return to honest subluxation-based patient care" and affordable fees, he stated:

> Unfortunately, some members of the chiropractic profession have been engaging in what amounts to "crime and wicked conduct" in their practices by jumping on the bandwagon of getting all they can from the insurance industry while the "getting" is good. They have been playing a numbers game of getting as many patient visits and as many dollars per visit by whatever means they (and often their practice management consultants) can devise. . . .
>
> Some members of our profession have been engaging in outright fraud with too many examinations and inflated office visit fees—which include inappropriate and often worthless therapies and x-ray procedures—that sometimes amount to $1,000 for the first visit before they've done anything at all for the patient! [266]

Daniel Futch, D.C., executive director of the National Association for Chiropractic Medicine, heads the chiropractic department of a large medical HMO in Wisconsin, where the law requires HMOs to include chiropractic services. Futch believes that if spinal manipulation cannot relieve a patient's symptoms within two weeks, additional manipulations are unlikely to help. He estimates that he and his associates see patients about half as often as the average chiropractor in private practice. Other Wisconsin chiropractors who regard such "low" utilization rates as a serious economic threat have lobbied for a law to force HMOs to hire more chiropractors, but so far they have not succeeded. In several other states, chiropractors are suing HMOs that do not include them.

Workers' Compensation

In trying to justify what they do, many chiropractors tout the findings of various workers' compensation (WC) studies. However, these studies did not scientifically validate what chiropractors do and were not designed for that purpose. Willem Assendelft, M.D., and Lex Bouter, Ph.D., have identified sixteen WC studies reported from 1966 through 1990 and analyzed them in the leading chiropractic journal [11]. Although most contain data appearing to favor chiropractic, Assendelft and Bouter concluded that "irreparable" methodological drawbacks make it impossible to draw trustworthy conclusions. Most of these reports lack detailed descriptions of the patient's problems, diagnoses, and clinical course. Nor did their authors evaluate whether patients going to chiropractors were comparable to those seeking medical care.

Without randomization, it stands to reason that people with the severest injuries will go to medical doctors and that the greater the injury, the more expensive the care will be. This is borne out by studies, cited by Assendelft and Bouter, which found that medical patients had more nerve-root involvement, greater back pain, and more initial disability than those going to chiropractors. Two studies they reviewed showed higher total treatment costs for chiropractic patients than for medical patients.

Assendelft and Bouter also noted that the duration and costs of disability and time lost from work are probably heavily influenced by factors other than effectiveness. Because the laws influencing compensation and health insurance vary from state to state, WC studies are unlikely to be comparable with one another or generalizable from one area of the country to another.

A recent federal report contains similar conclusions. In 1985, Congress directed the Department of Defense (DoD) to determine the cost-effectiveness of adding chiropractic care as a benefit for military families under its Civilian Health and Medical Program of Uniformed Services (CHAMPUS) program. The study project included a review of workers' compensation studies and an analysis of eighteen months' worth of data from a CHAMPUS demonstration project set up to compare the cost-effectiveness of chiropractic and medical care. The final report, issued in 1993, stated:

> Given current crises in health-care costs, and fiscal constraints within the military health care system, DoD does not favor inclusion of a benefit which cannot be justified with compelling evidence. To date, chiropractic studies have not produced such evidence. . . . Any requirement to establish these services under CHAMPUS should occur in the context of a managed care environment, should impose associated quality and utilization controls, and should be limited to services payable under Medicare. Only with strict controls . . . can the Department ensure delivery of care which is cost-effective, appropriate and medically necessary. [218]

Two chiropractors and a lawyer who studied WC data from Utah found the same methodological problems noted by Assendelft. They concluded that "issues of similarity in diagnosis and severity of the condition remain unanswered" and that "cost effectiveness of chiropractic care for industrial back-related injuries in Utah is not clearly established" [118]. The ACA's booklet "Chiropractic: State of the Art 1994–1995" conveniently omits these cautions while presenting data favoring chiropractic from the same report.

As with other programs of health-care reimbursement, there has been considerable chiropractic abuse of the WC system. During the late 1980s, undercover investigations by the Oregon State Workers' Compensation Fund resulted in the arrest of six chiropractors for allegedly falsifying an entire course of treatment [250]. Other chiropractors were found to be keeping two billing schedules—one for patients who paid out of their own pockets and another much higher price list for those covered by workers' compensation [89]. One man had more than one hundred chiropractic treatments, at a cost of more than $5,000, with no improvement. His problem turned out to be a ruptured disc fragment that required surgery. In 1990, in the wake of these events, Oregon's WC law was revised to limit chiropractors to twelve visits or thirty days of treatment per year, whichever came first.

In 1992, *Florida Trend* magazine published a cover story on "why chiropractors get blamed for fueling the cost of workers' compensation"

[54]. It describes unscrupulous chiropractors who abuse the system. Author Richard Coletti said, "Workers' compensation is fraught with abuse, but no other players in the system rile business more than the chiropractors." A spokesman for the American Insurance Association stated, "Sometimes I think of workers' comp as the chiropractic full-employment act." The main complaints were about exaggerated diagnoses, overtreatment, and aggressive marketing aimed at patient retention from cradle to grave. Coletti said that health-insurance companies have responded by calling for limits on chiropractic treatment, as had been imposed in Oregon. Some said they wanted chiropractors out of the WC system altogether.

Coletti's investigation turned up sweetheart relationships between chiropractors and lawyers:

> Less scrupulous attorneys turn to chiropractors, hoping they will give injured workers the highest impairment rating and extend treatment for as long as possible. The chiropractors who play the game are then rewarded with a steady stream of clients provided by their unspoken lawyer/partners.
>
> The payback for a lawyer comes in the medical expenses: The larger the expenses, the more the lawyer can expect, with legal fees paid by the insurer. . . . If a carrier disputes a claim . . . the lawyer can rack up hefty costs for time-consuming depositions and pre-trial appearances. Meanwhile, the chiropractor continues to provide treatment.

William P. Barrett, a writer for *Forbes* magazine, stumbled upon a similar arrangement in Albuquerque, New Mexico [26]. After a minor car accident, he was bombarded with letters and phone calls from half a dozen chiropractors who had obtained his name from an accident report. The messages suggested that he might have a hidden injury and offered a free examination and x-rays. Upon investigation, he found that one of these D.C.s steered his patients to a lawyer who would file a claim and push it through the insurance company. Then the attorney would pay the chiropractic bills after taking his cut from the insurance company's reimbursement. The patients did not have to pay anything. They just had to be insured.

In recent years, Medicare carriers and many insurance companies have instituted procedures whereby claims for more than twelve chiropractic visits are closely scrutinized. Unscrupulous practices have also led some employers to choose health plans that don't include chiropractic coverage. An attorney writing in a chiropractic journal warned of a "nationwide trend to reduce or eliminate access to chiropractic care for injured workers" [12].

The Bottom Line

Although some of the problems described in this chapter occur among other health practitioners, others are unique to chiropractic. Is it possible that pseudoscience and poor ethics go hand in hand?

11

The AMA Antitrust Suit

In 1976, Chester A. Wilk, D.C., and four other chiropractors initiated a federal lawsuit charging that the American Medical Association (AMA), the American Osteopathic Association, the American Hospital Association, the American College of Radiology, the Joint Commission on Accreditation of Hospitals, and several other organizations and individuals had engaged in an illegal boycott intended to destroy the chiropractic profession. Several more suits were filed against the AMA and others in state courts, and one suit was even filed by the New York Attorney General.

In each case, the defendants were accused of unreasonably restraining their members from developing professional relationships with chiropractors. The plaintiffs believed that since chiropractors were licensed, an organized attempt to destroy their profession would violate antitrust laws.

The defendants believed that their antichiropractic activities were justifiable because they were intended to protect the public. From the legal perspective, however, it was clear that the lawsuit would be expensive and might be difficult to win. If the courts ruled that chiropractic's shortcomings were irrelevant to antitrust law, the defendants might be defenseless. Under antitrust law, any damages awarded would be tripled and the loser might have to pay the winner's attorneys' fees—which, in this case, could be millions of dollars. Rather than face these risks, some of the organizations settled their cases with a pledge to terminate any interference with the right of their individual members to engage in professional cooperation with chiropractors.

137

The First Trial

The Wilk case came to trial in 1980. After hearing eight weeks of testimony, the jury concluded that the defendants were innocent. Two years later, however, an appeals court overturned this verdict and ordered a new trial on grounds that the original judge had misinterpreted the law. The appeals court ruled, in effect, that why the defendants campaigned against chiropractic was less important than whether their actions suppressed competition. The appeals court judges felt that "evidence tending to show that chiropractic is in fact quackery" might bear on the defendants' motives, but the "extravagant amount" introduced during the trial might have unfairly prejudiced the jury.

What evidence? Documents available from the record of the Wilk trial make it crystal clear why the AMA and its allies believed that something was drastically wrong with the chiropractic profession. For example:

• One document listed forty-eight reasons why chiropractors should obtain spinographs (14" x 36" full-spine films used to detect "subluxations"). The list had been published in a 1957 textbook by a "professor and lecturer of spinography and x-ray practice" at the Palmer College of Chiropractic. The reasons included:

    2 – It promotes confidence.
    4 – It creates interest among patients.
    6 – It reveals facts, chiropractically.
    7 – It produces business.
   10 – It attracts a better class of patients.
   11 – It builds prestige for you in the community.
   12 – It is the proper way to explain chiropractic.
   14 – It is the key to chiropractic success and health.
   15 – It reveals the vertebral misalignment.
   23 – It will reveal conditions which symptoms cannot.
   30 – It means the difference between chiropractic success and failure.
   31 – It helps to eliminate the so-called "starvation period" that many practitioners go through.
   32 – It provides a quicker way to build a chiropractic practice.
   35 – Its income makes it possible to arrange a better service.
   38 – It provides good interest on your investment.
   43 – It helps build unity in the chiropractic profession.

• Another document described how a Canadian professor of radiology visited three chiropractic schools during the early 1960s. Posing as the parent of a prospective student, he requested a tour of the facilities and asked about the training offered in x-ray procedures. At National College of Chiropractic:

> Our guide [a chiropractor] . . . took us to a room which contained an illuminator, a device used to view films. He took several films from an envelope and placed them on the illuminator—all upside down.
>
> The films showed a gallbladder filled with contrast drug and containing gallstones. Our guide, however, did not comment on the gallstones. Instead, he replaced the films with others which, he said would show a gallbladder. The films also were placed on the illuminator upside down.
>
> This second series of films showed a healthy gallbladder, but the chiropractor explained to us that "this is the gallbladder," at which point he sketched with his finger . . . a loop of intestine slightly distended with gas.
>
> Later on, we asked . . . who taught anatomy at the school and he replied, "I do."

• Project Hope (Health Opportunity by Periodic Examination) was advanced in 1974 by the Parker Chiropractic Research Foundation (PCRF), the leading chiropractic practice-building organization. The project's purpose was to persuade patients who had completed "their initial, intensive and corrective care" to continue chiropractic care for "maintenance and preventive benefits." The instructions—comprising ten pages— admonish PCRF's clients to: "REMEMBER – TRULY NO ONE IN THE WORLD SHOULD HAVE A CHIROPRACTIC ADJUSTMENT LESS OFTEN THAN ONCE A MONTH." For patients who balk at the cost of such lifetime care, the instructions recommend saying:

> Yes, I guess any amount of money is a lot of money, but it is all relative. . . . After all, what is life worth? What is health worth? What is just feeling good worth? What is being able to work worth? And what is being able to raise your family worth? Mr. Williams, you are really dealing now with your most priceless asset – your health. Yes, really your own life, so don't begrudge yourself this very necessary expenditure. Free nerve supply is as valuable as food.

The Second Trial

Before the Wilk case was retried, several more groups reached settlement agreements. The remaining parties agreed that the case would be decided by a judge rather than a jury, and the chiropractors relinquished their claims for financial damages. The second trial was held in the courtroom of United States District Court Judge Susan Getzendanner in Chicago. In 1987, Getzendanner dismissed four of the remaining defendants but ruled that the AMA and two other groups had violated the Sherman Antitrust Act [86]. A federal appeals court upheld this verdict, and the U.S. Supreme Court declined further consideration.

Getzendanner's lengthy opinion described how, during the early 1960s, the AMA had formed a committee on quackery whose primary objective was to contain and eliminate chiropractic as a form of health care. The committee sponsored conferences, helped prepare critical publications, and engaged in other activities intended to discourage professional association between medical doctors and chiropractors. In 1966, the AMA House of Delegates passed a resolution calling chiropractic an unscientific cult and declaring it unethical for physicians to associate professionally with chiropractors. In 1980, in an attempt to comply with antitrust laws, the AMA had revised its principles of medical ethics and replaced the above policy by declaring that physicians "shall be free to choose whom to serve, with whom to associate, and the environment in which to provide medical services." But Getzendanner ruled that this change was not sufficient to correct the damage done by the AMA's antichiropractic campaign. She concluded:

> The AMA had a genuine concern for scientific methods in patient care, and . . . this concern was the dominant factor motivating the AMA's conduct. However, the AMA failed to establish that throughout the entire period of the boycott, from 1966 to 1980, this concern was objectively reasonable. . . . The AMA's concern for scientific method in patient care could have been adequately satisfied in a manner less restrictive of competition. . . .
>
> None of the court's findings constituted a judicial endorsement of chiropractic. All of the parties to the case, including the plaintiffs, and the AMA, agreed that chiropractic treatment of diseases such as diabetes, high blood pressure, cancer, heart disease and infectious disease is not proper, and that the historic theory of chiropractic that there is a single cause and cure of disease was wrong. . . . There was evidence that the chiropractic theory of subluxations was unscientific, and evidence that some chiropractors engaged in unscientific practices.

Getzendanner noted that during the 1960s "there was a lot of material available to the Committee [the AMA Committee on Quackery] that supported its belief that all chiropractic was unscientific and deleterious." She also criticized chiropractors for taking too many x-rays, and stated that "the treatment of patients appears to be undertaken in an ad hoc rather than on a scientific basis."

The Current Situation

Although association with chiropractors is no longer considered unethical *per se*, most physicians have little respect for them. A 1993 American Chiropractic Association survey found that only 3 percent of chiropractors' patients were referred to them by a medical or osteopathic physician [47]. Another recent survey revealed that very few referrals were being made by HMO physicians [31].

Medical avoidance of the unscientific element in chiropractic has continued without urging by medical organizations. Until organized chiropractic jettisons all of its scientifically untenable theories and practices, few M.D.s will choose to work with chiropractors. Professional respect cannot be gained through a court order.

Chiropractic's relative isolation is imposed by its own deviant views of health and disease. How could self-respecting doctors cooperate with others who not only practice by a different paradigm (i.e., most disease is

In 1990, five weeks after the U.S. Court of Appeals upheld Judge Getzendanner's ruling, the American Chiropractic Association printed and distributed booklets containing its comments plus a complete copy of her opinion to more than 86,000 medical specialists, 40,000 magazine and newspaper editors, 9,000 college deans, 6,000 hospital administrators and trustees, 26,000 foundations that issue grants, and 65,000 chiropractors and students, as well as to members of Congress and state insurance commissioners, attorneys general, and supreme court judges.

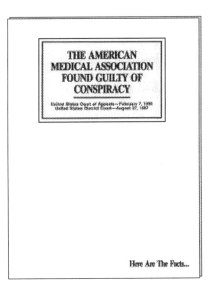

neurologically based) but also use a "different logic" [126]? Or who contradict medical science by disparaging proven surgical procedures, responsible drug therapy, and public health measures such as immunization, fluoridation of water, pasteurization of milk, and certain food-technology procedures?

Judge Getzendanner was careful to point out that her injunction "does not and shall not be construed to restrict or otherwise interfere with the AMA's right to take positions on any issue, including chiropractic, and to express or publicize these positions, either alone or in conjunction with others." Thankfully, some conscientious M.D.s are doing so, though they are reviled by chiropractic dogmatists and their hirelings. It would still be appropriate for the AMA to do what Getzendanner's verdict held to be reasonable: to mount a national educational program about chiropractic's shortcomings.

12

Deceptions Behind
Recent Headlines

As its hundredth anniversary approached, four reports about the treatment of low-back pain placed chiropractic in a favorable light. The first, referred to as the Meade study, was a British clinical trial that compared medical and chiropractic treatment [161]. The second, issued in several steps by the RAND Corporation, examined the appropriateness of spinal manipulation [223] [224] [225]. The third, produced by the Agency for Health Care Policy and Research (AHCPR), evaluated other treatments in addition to manipulation [33]. The fourth, produced for the Ontario Ministry of Health by health economist Pran Manga, Ph.D., and associates, compared the cost-effectiveness of chiropractic treatment and medical care [156].

Many chiropractors and members of the press have greatly magnified the significance of these reports. In 1991, for example, shortly after the Meade report was published, a prominent chiropractor discussed its findings on "CBS News Nightwatch." In response to the first RAND report, ABC's "20/20" gave favorable exposure, the *New York Times* printed a lengthy story headlined "Back Manipulation Gains Respectability" [206], and *Time* magazine published an article subheadlined "Once scorned as quackery, chiropractic is winning adherents and respect" [175]. According to the magazine article, the RAND report "found that chiropractic-style manipulation was helpful for a major category of patients with lower-back pain" and the Meade report had concluded that spinal manipulation by chiropractors was more effective than physical therapy. In 1994, after the AHCPR guidelines were issued, the Associated Press issued a story that began, "Chiropractors get a boost and surgeons a setback in a new

143

government-backed guidelines on how to treat low-back pain" and a chiropractic journal article even warned that failing to tell patients that manipulation is a treatment option could render physicians vulnerable to a malpractice suit for lack of "informed consent" [229]. The Manga report has generated considerable publicity in Canada. This chapter looks behind the headlines and examines what the reports actually mean.

The Meade Study

This British study, reported in the *British Medical Journal* in 1990, was a randomized controlled trial that compared hospital physical therapy with chiropractic treatment for low-back pain of mechanical origin. All five authors were medical practitioners. The study concluded:

> For patients with low back pain in whom manipulation is not contraindicated, chiropractic almost certainly confers worthwhile, long-term benefit in comparison with hospital outpatient management. The benefit is seen mainly in those with chronic or severe pain.

The study involved 741 patients between the ages of 18 and 65 who lacked signs of spinal nerve root compression, infectious disease, or other conditions that require medical intervention. The chiropractic treatment spanned up to 30 weeks (versus 12 weeks for hospital-based treatment) and cost about 50 percent more. The outcome was measured by a self-administered questionnaire about pain intensity, not a clinical evaluation. Patients with no prior history of back pain showed no difference in outcomes. Among patients with a prior history, those in the chiropractic treatment group scored significantly better than those in the hospital-based group at 6-, 12-, and 24-month follow-up intervals. The cost of treatment (1988–89 prices) averaged £165 per chiropractic patient and £111 per hospital treatment.

Although the authors cautioned that their findings "cannot be automatically applied to all patients with back pain," chiropractors have turned this study into a public-relations windfall. But they have deliberately failed to tell the whole story. The study does not prove that chiropractic is more effective than medical treatment for low-back pain. It was a "pragmatic" trial in which the type, frequency, and duration of treatment would be up to whoever was treating the patients. In other words, no treatment protocols were set up in advance to permit clear-cut comparisons. This experimental design has a significant disadvantage: If a difference is found between treatment types, it may not be possible to identify the components responsible for the difference. More important, although the study reflected how certain chiropractors treated patients, it did not reflect how they would normally decide which patients to treat. Nor is it possible to tell whether the treatments they administered were identical to those used in the United States.

The main criterion for eligibility was that patients had no problem for which manipulation would be dangerous. To determine this, all patients underwent a *medical* evaluation during which a hospital radiologist interpreted their x-ray films. Somewhere between 25 and 50 percent of otherwise eligible patients who were willing to enter the study were judged "ineligible" due to contraindications to manipulation. (The exact percentage can't be calculated from the published data because for many of these patients, the reason for ineligibility was not specified.) This is not what usually happens when patients go directly to chiropractors. As Dr. William T. Jarvis noted in a recent letter:

> The real value of any study is its applicability to the real world. . . .
> This study lost much of its applicability by screening patients
> carefully . . . accepting only those with no contraindications to
> manipulation. . . . There is no reason for anyone familiar with
> chiropractic practices to believe that similar screening is regularly
> done by most chiropractors. On the contrary, chiros are notorious
> for their overuse of manipulation, applying it for conditions for
> which there is no justification.

The study's methodology had several other significant flaws. Of those beginning the study, 14 percent missed treatments, did not complete the six-week questionnaire, or otherwise dropped out. The reasons for these withdrawals were not assessed, producing another variable that reduced the quality of the study. The evaluators who assessed treatment outcome (using straight leg raising and lumbar flexion tests) were not blinded to the treatment type, which may have biased the results. Most important, the authors noted that some of the physical therapists had such high caseloads that they "almost certainly . . . were unable to give all the specific treatment they would have wished to all patients." In contrast, the chiropractors, who were not included in the National Health Service, worked in private clinics. The chiropractic patients received 44 percent more treatments, with greater frequency and over twice as long a time span. It would have been more equitable to compare private physical therapists and private chiropractors so that the variable of undertreatment would have been eliminated. Dr. Meade and an associate recommended that further trials be done to identify which factors might have influenced the outcome of their study [162].

The authors estimated that of some 300,000 patients referred each year to a hospital for treatment of back pain, about 72,000 (24 percent) would be expected to have no contraindication to manipulation. This would mean that 76 percent of the patients seeking treatment at a hospital clinic would not be suitable for chiropractic treatment. It would be interesting to know what proportion of patients seeking treatment at chiropractic offices are unsuitable (by medical standards) and whether chiropractors advise them to go elsewhere.

The RAND Study

The RAND study is a project of the RAND Corporation, of Santa Monica, California, a highly respected nonprofit organization that does research in a variety of fields and maintains the largest non-university-based health sciences research center. The study was cosponsored by the UCLA School of Medicine, and funded by two chiropractic research organizations. The seven-member team that conducted it was led by Paul G. Shekelle, M.D., M.P.H., and included three chiropractors.

The overall project, titled "The Appropriateness of Spinal Manipulation for Low-Back Pain," has four parts. Stage I reviewed what is known about the effectiveness, complications, and indications for spinal manipulation for back pain. Its analysis was based on sixty-seven relevant articles and nine books published between 1955 and 1989 [225]. Stage II convened nine experts to evaluate when manipulation might be appropriate for low-back pain. Four of the nine panelists have chiropractic degrees [224]. Stage III repeated the study done in Stage II with a panel of nine chiropractors [223]. Stage IV, which has not yet been published, will judge the appropriateness of services rendered by a random sample of practicing chiropractors, with an emphasis on patients treated for low-back pain. So far, the principal findings have been:

- Data from twenty-two controlled studies support the use of manipulation for acute low-back pain in patients showing no signs of lower-limb nerve root involvement. However, only four of these studies involved manipulation by chiropractors.

- There was insufficient evidence to support the use of manipulation for most types of chronic back pain.

- Scientific reports provide no help in deciding when manipulative treatment should be stopped, with respect to either improvement or worsening of symptoms. It is not clear how many, if any, manipulations are necessary after a patient becomes pain-free.

• The frequency of complications from spinal manipulation for low-back pain had not been studied systematically. Although the risk appears small when compared to the large number of manipulations performed, no firm conclusions could be drawn because there were few data in the scientific literature.

• No published scientific evidence supports any of the treatment durations for different indications that have been proposed.

• The Phase II multidisciplinary panel concluded that out of 1,550 sets of possible circumstances, manipulation was appropriate for 112 (7 percent), inappropriate for 924 (60 percent), and equivocal for 514 (33 percent). [These figures do not mean that only 7 percent of patients with low-back pain should receive manipulation, since most of the problems within that 7 percent are much more common than many of the conditions represented by the other 93 percent. Furthermore, some exceptions are to be expected and practitioners of manipulation do have other treatments that may be appropriate for some of these other indications.] The Phase III chiropractic panel rated 1,570 indications and judged 27 percent appropriate, 48 percent inappropriate, and 25 percent equivocal [223].

• The appropriate indications for manipulation include: (a) low-back pain of less than three weeks' duration, (b) no or only minor neurologic findings (such as diminished ankle reflex), (c) no evidence of sciatic nerve root irritation (no shooting pain in the posterior thigh/calf or positive straight leg raising sign), and (d) no adverse response to prior manipulation [222].

• An appropriate trial of manipulation for low-back pain is two weeks for each of two different types of manipulation, after which, if there is no improvement, therapy should be discontinued.

• Inappropriate indications for manipulation include: (a) no response or an unfavorable response to prior spinal manipulation; (b) x-ray evidence of a malignant tumor, osteomyelitis, inflammatory arthritis, septic arthritis, or an acute or unhealed fracture; (c) no x-rays but the presence of risk factors such as fever, history of malignancy, severe osteoporosis, age greater than fifty, significant trauma, and the like; (d) pain of greater than six months duration; (e) prior operation on a vertebra in the area; (f) major neurologic findings; (g) lack of response to the current spinal manipulation; and (h) certain types of herniated disks [222].

Note that unlike the traditional chiropractic "subluxation," some of the above-mentioned conditions actually cause nerve-root impingement. B.J. Palmer and his disciples claimed that most diseases were caused by pinched nerves and could be remedied by spinal manipulation. How ironic that some types of actual "nerve compression" are a reason to *avoid* manipulation!

Chiropractic Distortions of RAND

Although chiropractors have promoted the RAND study as an endorsement of chiropractic, it is not. It merely supports the use of manipulation in carefully selected patients. Only a few of the reports identified by the RAND panel involved manipulation by chiropractors; most were done by medical doctors and physical therapists. Even more important, the RAND panel's conclusions about patient selection and treatment duration don't jibe with what takes place in chiropractic offices. Most chiropractors manipulate the vast majority of patients who walk through their door, some use manipulative techniques that have not been studied scientifically, and many urge all of their patients to undergo lifetime "preventive mainte-nance." In addition, many chiropractors emphasize a "dynamic thrust" technique, which is more vigorous (and therefore less safe) than the controlled manipulation used by other practitioners.

In an article titled "RAND Misquoted," published in the July 1993 *ACA Journal of Chiropractic*, Shekelle set the record straight by responding to six "common misinterpretations" of the RAND study and specifying what *had* been concluded (see box opposite). In a note preceding the article, an editor of the journal said, "The chiropractic profession should not and cannot afford to alienate a research organization of RAND's caliber, nor distort information resulting from its studies. In so doing, chiropractic undermines its own credibility." The note also criticized the International Chiropractors Association for advertising that the Meade and RAND studies "show the clinical effectiveness of chiropractic care."

Shekelle's letter was followed by pleas for accuracy and integrity when writing about research on manipulation. One was written by the president of the Foundation for Chiropractic Education and Research, and the other was written by John J. Triano, D.C., a well respected chiropractor who served on both the RAND and AHCPR expert panels. Nevertheless,

Excerpts from a Letter to the Chiropractic Profession from Paul G. Shekelle, M.D., M.P.H., RAND Corporation (1993)

Through RAND's process of monitoring the popular media, we have become aware of numerous instances where our results have been seriously misrepresented by chiropractors writing for their local paper or writing letters to the editor. RAND vigorously defends the integrity of its work, and we have had to write letters to these same newspapers pointedly correcting the misrepresentations. In order to avoid future similar embarrassments to the chiropractic profession, we would like to describe for your readers some common misinterpretations of our work.

• *The RAND Study showed that chiropractic is the most effective treatment for low-back pain.* RAND's results were about spinal manipulation, not chiropractic, and dealt with appropriateness, which is a measure of net benefits and harms. Comparative efficacy of chiropractic and other treatments was not explicitly dealt with.

• *The RAND study showed that chiropractic is the most cost-effective form of treatment for low-back pain.* Again, RAND's results are specific to spinal manipulation, and cost was specifically excluded from our analyses.

• *The RAND study showed that patients with low-back pain should first seek care from a doctor of chiropractic.* No mention is made from whom patients should seek care in our work.

• *The RAND study shows that chiropractic is the best form of care for many common musculoskeletal conditions.* We dealt only with low-back pain, and our results cannot be extrapolated to any other condition.

• *Any statement that links RAND research with care delivered to injured workers or workers' compensation.* We did not consider injured workers as a separate entity.

• *RAND showed that there is more good scientific evidence supporting chiropractic than there is for medical procedures.* Again, our work was specific to spinal manipulation, not the practice of chiropractic. It is true that there is more evidence to support the use of spinal manipulation as a treatment for some patients with low-back pain than there is for many medical procedures currently being used. It is not true that there is more evidence to support the use of spinal manipulation (or chiropractic) than there is to support the practice of medicine.

What *can* be concluded from RAND's research is:

• There is enough scientific evidence to justify the use of spinal manipulation for some patients with acute low-back pain.

• It is the judgement of a multidisciplinary group of back pain experts, based on the scientific literature and their clinical experience, that spinal manipulation is . . . appropriate . . . for some patients with low-back pain. [221]

A Review of Current Research

A Clinically and Cost-Effective Approach to Better Health

Chiropractic health care offers patients the advantages of a conservative, natural method of healing without the use of drugs or surgery. The primary form of treatment spinal manipulation or adjustment. For almost 100 years, patients have benefitted from chiropractic treatment. Recently, numerous studies have been published that support it effectiveness.

Chiropractic's Efficacy

Only about 15 percent of all medical interventions are supported by solid scientific evidence, according to David M. Edy, M.D., Ph.D., professor of health policy and management at Duke University, North Carolina.

In contrast, the breadth of existing research dedicated to chiropractic was noted by Paul G. Shekelle, M.D., MPH, of the RAND Corporation, on ABC's 20/20 when h said,"There are considerably more randomized controlled trials which show benefit of this (chiropractic) than there are for many, many other things which physicians and neurosurgeons do all the time."

Members of the Medical Community Recognize Chiropractic's Effectiveness

Shekelle, P.G., Adams, A., et al. *The Appropriateness of Spinal Manipulation for Lower-Back Pain.* RAND Corporation, Santa Monica, California, 1992:

This study conducted by the prestigious RAND Corporation marks the first time that representatives of the medical community have gone on record stating that chiropractic is an appropriate treatment for certain low-back pain conditions. A second, all-chiropractic panel's ratings show agreement with the multi-disciplinary panel that spinal manipulation is appropriate for specific kinds of low-back pain.

"The breadth of existing research dedicated to chiropractic was noted by Paul G. Shekelle, MD, MPH, of the RAND Corporation, on ABC's *20/20* when he said, 'There are considerably more controlled trials which show the benefit of this (chiropractic) than there are for many, many other things which physicians and neurosurgeons do all the time.'"

"The study conducted by the prestigious RAND corporation marks the first time that representatives of the medical community have gone on record stating that chiropractic is an appropriate treatment for certain low-back pain conditions."

The "review of current research" in the ACA's 1994–1995 "Chiropractic: State of the Art" booklet misrepresents the RAND study and Dr. Shekelle's "20/20" comments as endorsements for chiropractic. The word "this" in the "20/20" statement referred not to chiropractic but to spinal manipulative therapy [219].

the ACA's booklet "Chiropractic: State of the Art 1994–1995" misrepresents the RAND study as evidence of "chiropractic's efficacy" (see figure above), and so does a brochure published by the National Board of Chiropractic Examiners [242].

Such deceptive behavior does not surprise Dr. Jarvis. He believes that "most chiropractors appear to have only one criterion for evaluating a research report: its public relations value."

The AHCPR Guidelines

In December 1994, the Agency for Health Care Policy and Research (AHCPR), which is part of the U. S. Department of Health and Human Services, published a report called *Acute Low Back Problems in Adults*. It was the work of a twenty-three-member, multidisciplinary, private-sector panel that included two chiropractors. The panelists looked at published scientific studies and gave the greatest weight to randomized clinical trials. They did not consider back problems in children or problems that were considered chronic (present for more than three months).

The panelists considered manipulation a method of controlling symptoms while awaiting the spontaneous recovery that occurs within a month in up to 90 percent of patients with low-back problems. Other symptom-control methods include nonprescription pain-relievers, nonsteroidal anti-inflammatory drugs, muscle relaxants, oral steroid drugs, antidepressants, transcutaneous electrical nerve stimulation (TENS), shoe insoles and lifts, lumbar corsets and back belts, traction, and biofeedback. With respect to manipulation, the panel concluded:

> The evidence for effectiveness . . . varies depending on the duration and nature of the patient's presenting symptoms. For patients with acute low back symptoms without radiculopathy [nerve root dysfunction often caused by root compression], the scientific evidence suggests spinal manipulation is effective in reducing pain and perhaps speeding recovery within the first month of symptoms. For patients whose low-back problems persist beyond 1 month, the scientific evidence on effectiveness of manipulation was . . . inconclusive. For patients with radiculopathy, the scientific evidence was also inconclusive about either the effectiveness or the potential harms of manipulation. . . . For patients with acute low back problems and . . . possible progressive or severe neurologic deficits, assessment to rule out serious neurologic conditions is indicated before initiating manipulation therapy. [33:36]

As had the RAND group, the AHCPR panel evaluated spinal manipulation, not chiropractic. In fact, of the twelve well designed studies that the AHCPR panelists considered, only two involved chiropractors; and the

Part of brochure used to promote the ACA's "AHCPR kits."

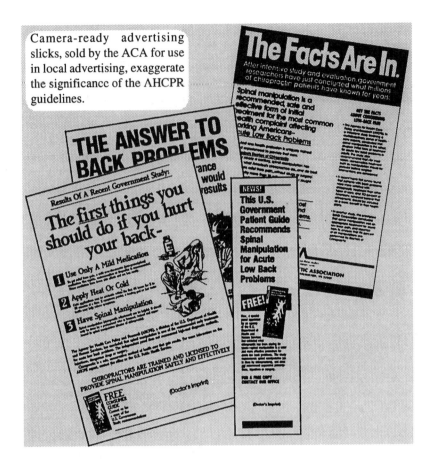

Camera-ready advertising slicks, sold by the ACA for use in local advertising, exaggerate the significance of the AHCPR guidelines.

word "chiropractic" does not actually appear in the text of the report. But chiropractors wasted no time in claiming that the report endorsed their work. The ACA informed its members that "the U.S. government has validated the effectiveness of spinal manipulation as it is done by chiropractors." For $49.50, members could purchase an "AHCPR Communications Kit" composed of ten copies of the clinical guidelines report, ten clinician quick-reference guides, one hundred consumer-version booklets, one hundred "patient thank you" pamphlets, and sample letters for contacting medical doctors, special interest groups, employers, industry executives, journalists, and managed-care leaders. ACHPR panel chairman Stanley J. Bigos, M.D., responded to the various promotions with a statement discouraging the use of "misrepresentations and . . . half-truths . . . for sensationalistic public relations value" [32].

The Manga Report

The Effectiveness and Cost-Effectiveness of Chiropractic Management of Low-Back Pain, commonly referred to as the Manga report, was written by Canadian economist Pran Manga, Ph.D., and three associates. The 104-page document, published in 1993, is based on their review of scientific publications and workers' compensation studies. The Ontario Ministry of Health funded the project in an effort to ascertain whether the rising costs of treatment for low-back pain might be contained by shifting resources from medical to chiropractic services. Its executive summary asserts that comparative data on effectiveness, cost-effectiveness, safety, and patient-satisfaction levels add up to "an overwhelming case" for much greater use of chiropractic services for low-back pain.

More effective? Manga's conclusions, like those of the RAND report, were based on studies of manipulative therapy. But the majority of these did not involve chiropractors.

More cost-effective? Manga's conclusions were based on workers' compensation studies. But, as pointed out in Chapter 10, the workers' compensation studies published so far have not been appropriately de-signed. So it is statistically improper to use them to estimate costs.

Safer? No valid comparison can be made about the safety of spinal manipulation because systematic studies have not been conducted.

Greater patient satisfaction? I don't doubt that many chiropractors have considerable ability to please their patients. (In fact, as noted else-where in this book, psychologically seductive techniques are taught by many chiropractic "practice-builders.") But patient satisfaction is influenced by many factors and does not necessarily mean that a treatment has been effective, cost-effective, or safe.

Nonetheless, in line with their dubious conclusions, Manga and associates recommended revamping Ontario's health-care system to foster the use of chiropractic services. Among other things: (a) chiropractic services should be fully insured, (b) health-care organizations should employ chiropractors, (c) hospitals should grant them full access to use their diagnostic and treatment facilities, (d) funds should be made available for further research into chiropractic management of low-back pain, (e) chiro-practic education should become university-based, and (f) chiropractors should be engaged at a senior level by the Workers' Compensation Board to assess policy, procedures, and treatment of workers with back injuries. As part of this last recommendation, the Manga report stated: "A very good case can be made for making chiropractors the gatekeepers for management of low-back pain in the workers' compensation system in Ontario."

Canadian chiropractors are using the Manga report in much the same way that American chiropractors have been using the AHCPR guidelines. They are advertising it as "government approval" and stressing its recommendation that chiropractors become "gatekeepers." An American Chiropractic Association lobbying kit makes the same suggestion [51].

Considering their inferior training and their propensity to overtreat, does the idea of chiropractors as gatekeepers appeal to you? It certainly makes no sense to me. Nor does the idea of forcing managed-care plans and hospitals to incorporate chiropractors into their programs. Integration into the medical mainstream cannot be forced or legislated. Chiropractic's isolation is self-imposed. Respectable scientists simply cannot work with pseudoscientists, no matter how many lawsuits or laws attempt to pressure them to do so. Chiropractic will never earn the respect of the medical profession unless it abandons Palmer's subluxation theory, opposition to immunization, and the multitude of dubious diagnostic and therapeutic procedures in which chiropractors are enmeshed.

Hamilton Hall, M.D., who is medical director of the Canadian Back Institute, director of the Spine Service at Toronto's Orthopaedic and Arthritic Hospital, and professor of surgery at the University of Toronto, has done a detailed analysis of the Manga report and identified many passages that are misleading and some that are factually incorrect [98]. Hall notes, for example, that while the Manga report implies that the University Hospital in Saskatoon is successfully using chiropractors as consultants, the actual situation involves chiropractic *students* who are mere *observers* and take no part in patient care or patient education [152]. Hall believes that the Manga report suffers from "a pervasive space bias, with anything positive to chiropractic given several paragraphs, while anything negative gets no more than a paragraph." Shekelle agrees that the Manga report is not well reasoned. In a recent note, he indicated that Manga had looked at the exact same studies as the RAND panelists, "but he is absolutely dead wrong on the cost-effectiveness conclusion and there are no data on relative safety" [220].

Do you wonder how Shekelle views chiropractic theory? In an interview published in 1992, he stated: "I don't for a second believe in what chiropractors call subluxations" [81]. And in a note published in the ACA journal that year, he stated: "Do the RAND reports prove the spinal subluxation theory of disease? . . . The answer . . . is . . . no" [226].

13

Research Considerations

Chiropractors maintain that their treatment "works." While some limit their practice to backaches and other musculoskeletal problems, others contend that their scope is unlimited. While some claim to increase the flexibility of joints—particularly those of the spine—others claim to restore the flow of "nerve energy" and/or "Innate Intelligence." As evidence of their effectiveness, chiropractors point to satisfied patients and a growing number of scientific studies and reports. This chapter examines the nature of chiropractic "research" and the validity of these claims.

The Trouble with Anecdotal Evidence

Let's begin by discussing why anecdotal evidence is not sufficient to establish that a treatment works. An anecdote is a report of personal observations not made under strict experimental conditions. A classic example is the story of the man who went to a chiropractor in the 1920s. After an examination, the patient was sent to the x-ray department. When he failed to return after an hour, the chiropractor phoned the department and was told that the man had left thirty minutes earlier. Two weeks later, the chiropractor received a letter from the man saying he was feeling much better now—thanks to that chiropractic x-ray treatment!

This story illustrates the natural human tendency to assume that if a health problem resolves following a course of treatment, the improvement is due to the treatment. To determine whether a treatment works, it is necessary to rule out coincidence, that is, whether the individual would have recovered just as well without it. This requires controlled experiments comparing people who receive the treatment with others (the "controls") who do not. Where anecdotes and testimonials are concerned, it is necessary to be sure that the events actually happened as claimed. The placebo effect should also be considered.

The Placebo Effect

The placebo effect is a beneficial change in a person's condition that occurs in response to a treatment but is not due to the pharmacological or physical aspects of the treatment. The therapeutic agent is usually a pill or a procedure. A patient need not believe in the placebo in order to feel better, but the effect is enhanced by faith and many other factors.

A striking example of the placebo effect was mammary artery ligation, a surgical procedure used in the 1940s and 1950s for treating chest pain (angina pectoris) due to coronary artery disease. Proponents believed that tying off the mammary arteries stimulated the growth of new blood vessels that would increase the supply of blood to the heart muscle. The procedure was considered effective until it underwent double-blind controlled tests. These remarkable studies demonstrated that pretending to operate but merely cutting the skin of the patient's chest wall was just as effective as tying off the mammary arteries [30].

In his landmark paper "The Powerful Placebo," Henry K. Beecher, M.D., observed that "for such subjective responses as pain . . . about a third of the affected people will respond to any placebo" [29]. Gordon Guyatt, M.D., and several colleagues added that "when an enthusiastic and trusted physician presents the interventions, the placebo response rate may increase to 70 percent" [92]. William T. Jarvis, Ph.D., states that the laying on of hands is likely to increase suggestibility, which enhances the placebo effect of spinal manipulative therapy [120]. Sympathetic attention, sensational claims (a tip-off that the treatment is a placebo), testimonials, and the use of elaborate and scientific-looking charts, devices, and terminology also promote the placebo effect. Research into spinal manipulation has found considerable placebo effect in the treatment of low-back pain. In one randomized, double-blind clinical trial, for example, 68 percent of patients receiving a sham manipulation reported an immediate reduction of pain [106].

The following true story illustrates how a chiropractor successfully used spinal manipulation as a placebo. During World War I, an American soldier developed shell shock. He became mute for over a year, until he went to a chiropractor back home who assured that a spinal adjustment would make him talk. Sure enough, immediately after the chiropractor adjusted the man's fifth cervical vertebra, he could talk. Since there was no physical reason for the muteness and since the cervical vertebrae have nothing to do with speech, this was clearly the power of suggestion coupled with placebo therapy used to treat hysterical muteness [255:216]. In this case it helped, but in most cases it is more appropriate for treatment to be provided by a trained psychologist or psychiatrist who can deal with the underlying emotional problems.

If spinal manipulation can relieve symptoms through a placebo effect, does this justify its use for that reason alone? The answer is no. Therapy should be based on the ability to alter abnormal physiology and not on the ability to elicit a less predictable placebo effect. Placebo therapy is inherently misleading and can make patients believe something is effective when it is not. As noted in Chapters 5 and 6, reformist Samuel Homola, D.C., warns that patients can become psychologically addicted to spinal manipulation [108] and that "by repeatedly demonstrating and treating imaginary subluxations of the vertebrae," the chiropractor "provides the patient with an ever-present 'cause' of disease and a constant fear of the position of his vertebrae" [107:96]. A further danger of placebo therapy is that it can validate and reinforce hypochondriasis. Moreover, placebos should be completely safe, and spinal manipulation is not.

Tests of manipulation should also take into account the fact that most people with back pain recover spontaneously within a few weeks [7] [253]. Without controlled clinical trials, any treatment that is used could receive credit for the body's natural recuperative ability.

Science or Pseudoscience?

Chiropractors have long insisted that chiropractic is a highly developed science. D.D. Palmer's 1910 textbook said that "Chiropractic is a proven fact—it is a science demonstrated by the art of adjusting" [181:876]. In his 1927 *Chiropractic Textbook*, R.W. Stephenson, D.C., reasoned that chiropractic was "a well developed science" because it fit a dictionary definition ("systematized knowledge considered as a distinct field of investigation or object of study")—a claim that has reverberated through chiropractic channels up to the present time. Although science fits this definition, so do medical astrology and virtually every other type of pseudoscience. As stated by Joseph C. Keating, Jr., Ph.D.:

Science is organized, systematized knowledge, but it is more. It is also the processes and activities scientists engage in, in order to collect and organize new knowledge and better applications. . . .

In order for chiropractic to develop as a science there must be a more widespread "opening of the chiropractic mind" and significant growth in chiropractic research activity. We must replace dogma with data, and we must let our most credible and systematic observations guide theory and practice in chiropractic. [130:4]

Keating is correct, but when valid research contradicts their dogma, chiropractors reject it. More than twenty years have elapsed since anatomist Edmund S. Crelin, Ph.D., demonstrated that the chiropractic "subluxation" does not pinch spinal nerves as they emerge between the vertebrae. Chiropractors contend that his test was not valid. But they have never conducted tests or produced contrary evidence obtained with x-rays, magnetic resonance imaging, or any other procedure which demonstrates that "pinching" of these nerves actually occurs. The American Chiropractic Association simply declares:

Chiropractic is based on three related scientific theories:
1. Pathological disease processes may be influenced by disturbances of the nervous system . . . .
2. Disturbances of the nervous system may be the result of derangements of the musculoskeletal structure. . . . The nerve compression hypothesis contends that aberrant neural activity results from mechanical disorders of the spine due to compression of spinal nerves at the intervertebral foramina. This hypothesis still occupies a central place in the chiropractic rationale.
3. Disturbances of the nervous system may aggravate pathological processes in various parts or with various functions in the body. [46]

These sentences are little more than a restatement of B.J. Palmer's "subluxation" theory using contemporary medical verbiage. They are certainly too vague to qualify as scientific hypotheses. Moreover, the words themselves (particularly the word "may" in all three items) confirm that chiropractic is founded upon something that *may not* exist.

In an attempt to excuse their lack of scientific support, chiropractors often cite a 1978 report by the Office of Technology Assessment which said that "only 10 to 20 percent of procedures currently used in medical practice have been shown to be efficacious by controlled trial" [173]. This citation is misleading for two reasons: First, since the report was published, the percentage of medical treatments validated by controlled trials has increased. Second, most of the rest have a logical basis and are supported by published studies based on careful observations. Most chiropractic procedures are supported by little more than wishful thinking.

Appropriate Testing of Spinal Manipulation

How can procedures be validated? The scientific method involves setting up testable hypotheses that can be shown to be either true or false. With respect to chiropractic, a suitable hypothesis might be, "Chiropractic spinal manipulation is effective for relieving chronic low-back pain of mechanical origin." This can be tested with randomized clinical trials (RCTs) which, ideally, should have the following characteristics.

- Patients must have back pain of comparable duration, severity, and type. There should be treatment and control groups large enough to enable detection of significant effects. The smallest group should have at least fifty patients. Assignment to the groups should be done randomly. Patients should be unable to tell which group they are in. This can be achieved by using patients who are unfamiliar with manipulation or who receive some type of "sham" manipulation.

- The type and number of manipulations per patient should be tabulated. Other treatments should not be administered simultaneously so that the chiropractic manipulation itself is the only therapy tested.

- There should be a low withdrawal rate during the trial, and dropouts must be accounted for.

- Outcome should be assessed by both the patients and an evaluator who does not know what therapy any patients received. The assessments should include pain relief, functional status, spinal mobility, overall improvement, and the need for drugs. Proper statistical analysis must be done.

This type of research is expensive and demanding. The chiropractic profession has done very little such work. Dutch researchers Bart W. Koes and his colleagues were able to locate and evaluate thirty-five clinical trials of spinal manipulation, but only six involved chiropractors [139]. Paul G. Shekelle, M.D., and colleagues reviewed twenty-five randomized controlled trials (RCTs), only four of which involved chiropractors and all of which were medically designed [227]. Thus the leaders in research on manipulation have been medical and osteopathic physicians and physical therapists, not chiropractors.

Little Significant Research

Chiropractors have a long tradition of scientifically invalid research. Sociologist Walter I. Wardwell, Ph.D., states that B.J. Palmer created the B.J. Palmer Chiropractic Clinic at his school in 1935 to carry out research on chiropractic, but that "true randomization and statistical controls were not used (and probably not even considered!)" [255:187]. William Heath Quigley, D.C., a Palmer faculty member, has admitted:

> Unfortunately, as a research facility it contributed very little. The principal reason for this failure was the total lack of qualified research personnel. The avowed goal was to prove that chiropractic adjustments reversed disease processes but the research design was fundamentally flawed. It was essentially this: each patient was examined once a week. These included blood tests, EKGs, CBCs [complete blood counts], urine tests, contourograms, etc. All these data were collected as if in a basket. . . . In 1951 an effort was made to extract some meaningfulness from the imposing collection. A statistically naive staff member made a well-intentioned effort, but there was not one mathematically valid technique for the testing of the significance applied and there were no controls. [202]

During the 1940s and 1950s, the few who advocated a vigorous program of chiropractic research gave it up as a hopeless cause, lamenting that even the chiropractic colleges would do nothing about it. Cultism was seen as the biggest deterrence to scientific research, and it still is. Keating, a research expert who contributes regularly to chiropractic journals, blames chiropractic's retarded scientific development on the persistence of chiropractic metaphysics [128].

Most chiropractic journals, magazines, and newspapers still reflect this lack of good science. Keating laments that "the trade magazines in chiropractic are replete with claims for experimentally unstudied methods (and for the value of unspecified chiropractic care)" [130:10]. Craig F. Nelson, D.C., calls some of the articles "chiro-babble," citing one on how to identify homicidal tendencies in a patient by means of x-ray analysis and another that used chiropractic principles to conclude that "AIDS is . . . non-infectious and cannot be transmitted sexually" [170]. Mitchell Haas, D.C., provided another glimpse into the shoddy nature of chiropractic research when he reviewed studies of the reliability of chiropractic procedures that had been published in peer-reviewed chiropractic journals between 1979 and 1990. He concluded that only ten out of forty-five had "properly supported conclusions" [93].

The most prominent example of futile chiropractic-sponsored research was probably that of Chung Ha Suh, Ph.D., a University of Colorado engineering professor who received support from the International Chiropractors Association plus a federal grant to study the biomechanics of "subluxations." Suh worked for more than ten years on computer models of spinal movement and spinal x-ray analysis. He reported on his activities at many ICA-sponsored conferences, but produced nothing that appears to have influenced chiropractic theory or practice in any way. In 1976, Scott Haldeman, D.C., Ph.D., M.D., justifiably criticized Suh for "attempting to find more accurate ways of measuring a subluxation in the absence of any solid data that a subluxation is worth measuring" [95]. In 1987, Jarvis added: "Although providing chiropractic public relations personnel with fodder for a decade, Suh's work on the elusive subluxation never got anywhere and now seems fruitless at best" [120]. Suh's work is not mentioned in the sections on biomechanical imaging of the spine in Haldeman's 1992 textbook [96].

The Medline database, which encompasses more than 3,600 biomedical journals, includes only one from chiropractic, the *Journal of Manipulative and Physiological Therapeutics* (JMPT). In 1989, Keating surveyed JMPT's first thirty-six issues (1978–1986) and reported that only three out of 334 papers described controlled clinical trials of chiropractic methods [132]. Since that time, the quality and publication rate of controlled studies have increased considerably, but their findings appear to have little effect on chiropractic practice. There is no evidence, for example, that studies debunking the muscle-testing procedure of applied kinesiology have caused its popularity to decline.

This is an extremely important point. Research findings in major medical journals can have enormous impact on what physicians do. Moreover, new drugs must undergo extensive scientific testing in order to gain FDA approval for marketing, and adverse reactions are reported to medical journals and the FDA. *Nothing parallel to this exists within chiropractic.* Whereas medical journals are widely read by physicians, chiropractic journals have few subscribers (fewer than 10 percent subscribe to JMPT, for example). Many chiropractors read no journals at all. And cherished chiropractic beliefs tend to be rigidly held.

The Bottom Line

Although several chiropractic colleges have developed what Keating appropriately calls "serious intellectual subcultures" [129] and much research is now under way, "chiropractic science" is still in its infancy. Very little has been done to sort out the pros and cons of the over two hundred chiropractic manipulation techniques that have been described. Very little is known about the frequency with which manipulation should be used to treat neuromuscular problems. Almost nothing has been done to determine whether any other ailments fall within chiropractic's legitimate scope. Little or nothing has been done to evaluate the dozens of questionable diagnostic and therapeutic procedures described in Chapters 7 and 8 of this book. No systematic survey of large numbers of patients has been done to determine the rates of chiropractic injuries, even though the sparse data from chiropractic malpractice insurers indicate that a comprehensive study is needed.

Of course, if any of this is done, it remains to be seen whether it will influence how chiropractors think and act.

14

Significant Risks Remain

Of all the half-truths and false assertions of chiropractors, the most serious is the assurance that their manipulations are safe. Chiropractic's other misrepresentations merely invite people to waste time and money. This one invites people to waste their health and even their life!

The most serious complication of spinal manipulation is a cerebrovascular accident ("stroke") caused by rupture of an artery to the brain. It can occur because the arteries that thread through the cervical vertebrae can tear when suddenly shifted by manipulation of the neck.

One person who suffered a stroke is Tina Frazier, whom I mentioned briefly in Chapter 1. Tina is a soft-spoken mother of two young children. Like many other survivors of chiropractic complications, she required

Right-sided view of the cervical (neck) vertebrae and the right vertebral artery. The vertebral arteries, one on each side, thread through holes in the six upper cervical vertebrae. Sudden rotation of the neck can injure these arteries and interrupt the flow of blood to the lower part of the brain.

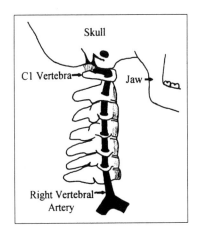

professional help to deal with feelings that she was deceived, exploited, injured, and deserted by a licensed health professional. Here's what she wrote to me:

> There had been no warning. Before I knew it I had blacked out. When I came to, I had double vision and was *paralyzed!!* The chiro called a neurologist, but did not listen to the physician's advice. Instead of being taken to a hospital, I was left in the office for over four hours. The chiro told me that I had only suffered a detached retina and that the paralysis was just a stress reaction. He still denies that I suffered a brain stem stroke, or that it was caused from having my neck manipulated.

The malpractice lawsuit filed by Tina was settled out of court with the chiropractor's insurer paying about $30,000 plus court costs. The arbitrator of the case concluded that the chiropractor had: (a) failed to take an adequate history, (b) failed to provide information needed for informed consent, (c) not kept complete records on her case, (d) failed to adequately consider the significance of her presenting symptoms, (e) allowed an unlicensed assistant to manipulate her neck, (f) not properly supervised his assistant, (g) continued to manipulate Tina's neck after she showed symptoms of an oncoming stroke, and (h) unduly delayed getting her to a hospital for the anticoagulation therapy desperately needed to reduce the severity of her stroke. The expert medical care she received was the only thing that helped her recover almost fully and kept the insurer's payment as low as it was. Tina got nothing for pain and suffering.

Another tragic case involves the late Sally A. Kaplan. Peter J. Modde, D.C., has described what happened as related by the attorney who handled her case:

> Sally . . . a 26-year-old housewife and new mother, entered a chiropractic office with her six-week-old daughter and requested treatment for a stiff neck that had been interfering with her breast-feeding and normal household activities. . . .
>
> The chiropractor did brief motion tests, but did not take any X-rays or perform any neurological examination. . . . He placed her in . . . face-up position on his adjusting table, placed his hands on opposite sides of her head, and twisted her neck, first left and then right. Immediately following the adjustment, Ms. Kaplan complained to the chiropractor that she could not "see straight" and was experiencing nausea and extreme headache. She was unable to raise her body from the table, and the chiropractor immediately called an ambulance. She was hospitalized within four hours of the adjustment and died the next morning [164:322].

How many people suffer the devastation of stroke from chiropractic manipulation each year? The vast majority of malpractice cases against chiropractors are settled out of court, often with a nondisclosure agreement to minimize public-relations damage to the profession. Speculations exist that the odds of a serious complication due to neck manipulation are somewhere between one in four hundred thousand and one in ten million. No one really knows, however, because: (1) as the RAND study pointed out, "There has been no systematic study of the frequency of complications from spinal manipulative therapy" [225]; and (2) the largest malpractice insurer appears reluctant to reveal what it knows.

Conflicting Data

The National Chiropractic Mutual Insurance Company (NCMIC) insures about half the chiropractors in the United States. Its brochure, *Chiropractic Malpractice Insurance . . . Plus,* promises potential clients that it will provide "a powerful legal network" behind them. The company also says that "approximately one in twenty chiropractors currently is involved in an active malpractice claim. And that figure is rising." NCMIC's Spring 1991 newsletter, *Back Talk,* lists the following injuries and the percentage of total cases in which the company issued payment in 1990:

Bone fracture	21 percent
Cerebrovascular accident	20 percent
Disk rupture	19 percent
Failure to diagnose	18 percent
Vicarious	11 percent
Soft tissue injury	8 percent

Reformist Daniel Futch, D.C., executive director of the National Association for Chiropractic Medicine, contacted NCMIC by phone to obtain the actual number of strokes that 20 percent represented and was told that the company paid about seven hundred claims in 1990. That would mean that about 140 claimants for damages due to stroke had been awarded money either in court or, more commonly, in an out-of-court settlement. Although Futch and a colleague requested written confirmation repeatedly, they did not receive it. In 1995, I also wrote and received no reply.

Consumer Reports cited the figure of 140 in the article on chiropractors in its June 1994 issue. Afterward, however, NCMIC notified the magazine's editors that the actual number had been only twenty out of a total of 272 claims [91]. Something doesn't add up, because 20 percent of 272 is fifty-four. Assuming that chiropractors not insured by NCMIC produced an equivalent number of strokes, the national total for 1990 would be 40, 108, or 280, depending on which figure was accurate. The 108 figure is corroborated by a report from Timothy Perdian, D.C., that in 1989, NCMIC had paid out forty-nine claims for stroke [188]. Malpractice settlements, of course, don't present the full story. Most victims of professional negligence do not take legal action. Even when serious injury results, some are simply not inclined toward suing, some don't blame the practitioner, some have an aversion to lawyers, and some can't find an attorney willing to represent them [148] [163] [174:135].

In 1992, researchers at the Stanford Stroke Center asked 486 California members of the American Academy of Neurology how many patients they had seen during the previous two years who had suffered a stroke within twenty-four hours of neck manipulation by a chiropractor. The survey was sponsored by the American Heart Association. One hundred seventy-seven neurologists reported treating fifty-six such patients, all of whom were between the ages of twenty-one and sixty. One patient had died, and forty-eight were left with permanent neurologic deficits such as slurred speech, inability to arrange words properly, and vertigo. The usual cause of the strokes was thought to be a tear between the inner and outer walls of the vertebral arteries, which caused the arterial walls to balloon and block the flow of blood to the brain. Three of the strokes involved tears of the carotid arteries [144]. In 1991, according to circulation figures from *Dynamic Chiropractic*, California had about 19 percent of the chiropractors practicing in the United States, which suggests that about 147 cases of stroke each year were seen by neurologists nationwide. Of course, additional cases could have been seen by other doctors who did not respond to the survey.

Louis Sportelli, D.C., NCMIC president and a former ACA board chairman contends that chiropractic neck manipulation is quite safe. In an 1994 interview reported by the Associated Press, he reacted to the American Heart Association study by saying, "I yawned at it. It's old news." He also said that other studies suggest that chiropractic neck manipulation results in a stroke somewhere between one in a million and one in three million cases [100]. The one-in-a-million figure could be correct if California's chiropractors had been averaging about sixty neck manipulations per week. Later that year, during a televised interview with "Inside Edition," Sportelli said the "worst-case scenario" was one in five hundred thousand but added: "When you weigh the procedure against any other procedure in the health-care industry, it is probably the lowest risk factor of anything." According to the program's narrator, Sportelli said that 90 percent of his patients receive neck manipulation.

How significant are these numbers? The authors of the Stanford study describe the risk as "small but significant." *Consumer Reports* calls them significant. Considering the benign, self-limiting physical problems for which neck manipulation is used and the fact that some people who have neck manipulations for "preventive maintenance" have nothing wrong with them, I would call even *one* stroke significant.

In stark contrast to chiropractic, the medical profession diligently compiles information on adverse events. Accredited hospitals have standing committees to monitor many types of complications. Individual cases and statistical tabulations are reported at educational meetings and in medical journals. Adverse reactions to drugs and medical devices are also reported to the FDA, which watches for significant trends. Chiropractors are fond of pointing out that there are more complications due to treatment by medical doctors than there are from chiropractors. This argument is not legitimate, however, since the conditions treated are not comparable. Though some chiropractors aspire to treat much more, the scientifically valid scope of chiropractic practice involves musculoskeletal problems that are self-limiting and relatively benign. Most medical doctors treat problems that are more serious.

Delayed Strokes

The figures above, distressing as they are in terms of personal tragedies, do not take into account the accumulating evidence that strokes from neck manipulation are sometimes delayed for days or weeks [159]. Perdian suggests that when symptoms are not immediate, many victims fail to make a connection between the manipulation and their stroke. Furthermore, case studies suggest that the very neck or occipital (base of the skull) pain that can prompt fatal neck manipulation can be caused by previous vertebral artery injury, whether from chiropractic treatment, other trauma, or spontaneous.

In one such case, pathologist Michael R. Sherman, M.D., described what he observed during the autopsy of a chiropractic patient who died of a stroke:

> Examination of the right vertebral artery clearly indicated that it had been subjected to significant prior trauma, most likely as a result of the initial series of cervical manipulation. . . . The left vertebral artery exhibited what we believe to be the early . . . lesion, which, given time and repeated trauma in the form of manipulation, could evolve into a [condition] identical to that of the severely

compromised right vertebral artery. . . . It appears, in this case, that the prior manipulation the subject had undergone was the most significant and, indeed, the sole risk factor for subsequent [stroke]. . . . This study indicates that significant pathologic changes that may not be immediately apparent . . . occur in vertebral arteries. [228]

Neurologist Jean-Louis Mas, M.D., has warned that pain that precedes and motivates chiropractic cervical manipulation may be the first symptom of a dissecting aneurysm, a condition in which the interior of an artery wall is split and blood fills and enlarges the space, causing narrowing of the artery. In such a case, cervical manipulation would precipitate a stroke either by causing the blood-filled wall to further block the arterial passageway or by dislodging a blood clot which is carried to the brainstem [158].

These reports caution that rather than indicating a need for neck manipulation, some neck or occipital pain is actually a reason to avoid it!

Contraindications to Manipulation

Despite the assurance of Sportelli and other chiropractors that stroke following manipulation occurs predominantly in patients with predisposing factors, most reported cases reveal none [80] [228]. Nevertheless, many factors still can make neck manipulation unwise. The RAND report (see Chapter 12) mentions malignant tumors, osteomyelitis (bone infection), inflammatory arthritis, septic arthritis, and fracture of the spine.

A prominent chiropractic textbook contains an entire chapter on cerebrovascular complications of manipulation, written by Australian chiropractic educators Allen G.J. Terrett and Andries M. Kleynhans, D.C. Their list of general risk factors for vascular injury includes cigarette smoking, atherosclerosis, the use of anticoagulants or oral contraceptives, hypertension, diabetes, bony outgrowths, cardiovascular disease, headaches, whiplash, and a history of neck sprain. They stress that people who have transient ischemic attacks (TIAs)—spells characterized by dizziness, nausea, vomiting, lack of balance, disturbed speech, double vision, difficulty swallowing, and/or headache—should not be manipulated and may require immediate medical evaluation for impending stroke. They warn, however:

It does not appear that any of [these] factors, either alone or in combination, specifically increase susceptibility, as vascular injury does not appear to be related specifically to any age group or sex. It would be imprudent, however, to totally ignore the presence of one or more significant factors that indicate possible predisposition to accidents. [245]

Although some chiropractors perform "screening tests" with the hope of detecting individuals prone to stroke due to neck manipulation, these tests are not particularly effective. Listening over the neck arteries with a stethoscope to detect a murmur, for example, has not been proven reliable, though patients that have one should be referred to a physician. Vascular function tests in which the patient's head is briefly held in the positions used during cervical manipulation are also not reliable as a screen for high-risk patients. Terrett and Kleynhans state that "an accident may still occur because this test in no way is a predictor as to whether or not a thrust [which further stretches the vertebral artery] could damage the vessel wall." The vascular function tests themselves can induce a stroke. Terrett and Kleynhans conclude:

> Even after performing the relevant case history, physical examination, and vertebrobasilar function tests, accidents may still occur. There is no conclusive, foolproof screening procedure to eliminate patients at risk. Most victims are young, without [bony] or vascular pathology, and do not present with vertebrobasilar symptoms. The screening procedures described cannot detect those patients in whom [manipulation] may cause an injury. They give a false sense of security to the practitioner.

Several medical reports have described chiropractic patients who, after neck manipulation, complained of dizziness and other symptoms of transient ischemic attack, only to be remanipulated and have a full-blown stroke. During a workshop at the 1995 Chiropractic Centennial Celebration, Terrett said such symptoms are ominous and that chiropractors should abandon rotational manipulations that overstretch the vertebral arteries.

Benefit/Risk Assessment for Neck Manipulation

The standard way to evaluate a medical treatment is to compare its potential benefits with its possible harms. To gain permission to market a new drug, for example, the manufacturer must present evidence to the FDA that the drug will do far more good than harm in most situations in which it is used.

Few types of chiropractic treatment have been subjected to any sort of systematic benefit/risk assessment. However, National Association for Chiropractic Medicine president Charles E. DuVall, Jr., D.C., believes that the risk of serious harm from neck manipulation involving rotation and extension—even if it is rare—far outweighs the possible benefit. Many of the reported strokes were caused by treatment for such relatively minor and self-limiting problems as a stiff neck, neck-muscle pain, or headache, or even for "preventive maintenance" where the patient was completely healthy and pain-free. Some of these strokes probably involved treatment that had no realistic chance of relieving the problem at hand, such as neck manipulation for low-back pain, allergies, high blood pressure, acne, or head colds. Remember, too, that the few controlled trials on the efficacy of neck manipulation for the relief of pain have not produced conclusive findings [139] and that safer therapies are available for some of the problems for which chiropractors commonly use such manipulation.

National Council Against Health Fraud president William T. Jarvis, Ph.D., a leading consumer advocate in the health field, maintains that the dynamic thrust (a sudden, forceful maneuver) poses unacceptable risks of stroke and paralysis when used on the neck [122]. He advises: "Do not allow *anyone* to forcefully manipulate your neck under any circumstances!" Perdian states pointedly, "Cervical adjustments are dangerous. Any risk at all is too great a risk" [188]. Modde says that use of the rotation and extension technique on patients who are lying face up is "consistently dangerous, often lethal" and "constitutes blatant malpractice and cruel disregard for patients" [164:98].

DuVall and three colleagues are trying to develop a reliable screening procedure to identify patients who are predisposed to stroke from cervical manipulation [70]. Their first step was a pilot study of eleven healthy, symptom-free volunteers who were not in the proposed high-risk category (i.e., no history of TIAs, nonsmokers, no recent neck trauma, no vascular disease). Five of the eleven developed abnormal EEG readings when they voluntarily rotated and extended their neck, which meant that their vertebral artery blood flow was decreased. Four of these five had a history of neck injury. This finding may be important because it suggests that a history of neck injury, rather than indicating a need for neck manipulation involving extension and rotation (as many chiropractors would assume), is actually a contraindication.

Other Physical Risks

Another of the serious complications possible from chiropractic spinal manipulation is that of intervertebral disk rupture. In 1989, NCMIC reported 235 losses due to disk injuries [188]. Chiropractic "subluxations" do not compress the major nerves exiting the spine, but ruptured disks often do, causing severe, persistent pain in the back or neck that radiates down the arm or leg served by the injured nerve. Compression of spinal nerves has never been shown to cause visceral disease, but it is known to cause muscle weakness, loss of reflexes, and numbness. In extreme cases, manipulation of already damaged lumbosacral disks has resulted in cauda equina syndrome, which, in addition to back pain and weakness and numbness in the legs, involves urinary retention, bowel incontinence, numbness in the buttocks and genitalia, and impotence.

A large survey of back-pain sufferers conducted in the early 1980s found that chiropractic treatment of acute pain from ruptured disks worsened the condition in 29 percent of the cases and that chiropractors were more prone than other practitioners to cause increased pain [136:242]. The RAND report also states that spinal manipulation has not been shown to reduce disk herniation [225:8].

Modde's book, *Chiropractic Malpractice,* lists other risks of spinal manipulation. Among them are spinal cord damage, cardiac arrest, arthrosis (joint degeneration), and permanent joint damage. The last of these is related to the problem of overadjusting. Chiropractors are notorious for pushing long-term spinal adjusting schedules on their patients. Intense and frequent manipulation is not only unnecessary, it can also be harmful. Modde writes: "After the initial care, that is on the average after ten to twenty treatments . . . the treatment itself can actually work as an irritant and perpetuate the original condition" [164:245]. He suggests that by frequently adjusting their patients' spines, some chiropractors are creating their own marketplace.

For three years during the late 1960s, Michael Livingston, M.D., a family physician who practiced in Canada and specialized in manipulation, examined 676 patients who had undergone spinal manipulation. He concluded that twelve out of the 172 who had visited a chiropractor during their lifetime had been harmed—some from undue force, and others due to misdiagnosis [147]. The techniques he reported (such as jumping from a stool onto a patient's back and "judo-chopping" a patient's neck) may not be practiced today, but Livingston's report is interesting nonetheless. In 1992, California neurologists who responded to the American Heart Association's survey reported seeing forty-six cases of nerve or muscle injury in addition to the fifty-six strokes mentioned above [144].

Many chiropractors advertise that people with whiplash injuries should consult them. Some furnish conservative treatment, while others manipulate the neck. However, Meridel I. Gatterman, D.C., who has been director of chiropractic sciences at two chiropractic colleges, states that the sprained and strained areas involved in whiplash injury should not be manipulated [82:60].

Samuel Homola, D.C., warns that since vigorous thrusting "often forces the joint slightly beyond its range of normal movement.... Repeated, unnecessary manipulation of a normal spine joint would probably place a strain upon the ligaments holding the joint together, and further put the intervertebral disk fibers through stresses they do not usually receive." He adds that "a joint once strained excessively in its ligamentous structure is not thereafter a thoroughly strong joint. A ligament cannot be rehabilitated like a muscle" [107:43]. The prominent orthopedist Ruth Jackson, M.D., agrees. She states that if the ligamentous and capsular structures of the joints are subjected to a deforming force beyond their functional capacity, they do not regain their original length when the deforming force is removed [115:120]. Overadjusting a vertebrae can result in permanently stretched ligaments, causing chronic instability so that the adjustments no longer "hold," thus necessitating periodic readjustments of the same vertebrae. As noted in Chapter 12, RAND's expert interdisciplinary panel recommended that an appropriate trial of manipulative therapy would be only two weeks of treatment for each of two different types of manipulation [224:91].

The Risk of Misdiagnosis

Chapter 4 points out the shortcomings in chiropractic education past and present. Although chiropractic education has certainly improved during the past fifteen years, most chiropractors have not learned the fine points of differential diagnosis, and in some situations they are not legally permitted to perform the tests necessary to reach appropriate conclusions. A few chiropractors even maintain that their role is to diagnose "subluxations" rather than disease. Because of this, people who use a chiropractor as a primary-care physician incur the risk of a failure to get either appropriate care or a referral for such treatment, especially for serious diseases that may *appear* to be of musculoskeletal origin but are not.

Many tragic examples could be given of people who went to chiropractors and were treated by spinal manipulation while an undetected illness progressed beyond remedy of the proper medical treatment. Wallace I. Sampson, M.D., a cancer specialist in Santa Rosa, California, for example, says he has seen more than a dozen people with undiagnosed cancer who were damaged by chiropractic spinal manipulation [27]. Even in the arena of musculoskeletal problems, diagnostic chaos is common, as shown by numerous investigations where the same individual, examined by several chiropractors, received different diagnoses from most of them [21].

Chiropractors, of course, do not have a monopoly on diagnostic failure. Medical doctors make many mistakes too, but their failure is not usually the result of inadequate training or a "philosophy" that clouds their thinking. John Badanes, D.C., a scientifically oriented chiropractor in Berkeley, California, believes that most chiropractors should not even be considered competent musculoskeletal doctors (or "back specialists"), since the clinical training in most chiropractic schools has emphasized "finding and fixing subluxations," which is a delusional pursuit. Modde has warned:

> The more the patient relies on the chiropractor for diagnosis . . . the more vulnerable he will be. Patients who use chiropractors as primary physicians, either because they don't know any better or because they have been turned off by orthodox medical care, run the greatest risk. [165]

Unnecessary Radiation

Ionizing radiation is potentially dangerous because it increases the likelihood of developing certain cancers. In addition, x-ray exposure of women who later bear children can increase the prevalence of birth defects in future generations. This is not reason to avoid diagnostic x-rays altogether, because there are many situations where they yield valuable information. Responsible practitioners restrict the use of diagnostic x-rays to situations where the potential benefit outweighs the likelihood of harm.

More than twenty years ago, for example, the medical profession stopped recommending routine chest x-rays because the likelihood of finding a treatable condition in patients with no symptoms was considered smaller than the likelihood of harm from the radiation involved. Chiropractic spinography (done with 14" by 36" x-ray films) exposes patients' sexual organs to between ten and one thousand times as much radiation [20]. Ted Fickel, D.C., Ph.D., has calculated that a full-spine examination in a young adult with no symptoms is more likely to cause a bony cancer than to detect one [76]. Concerning the genetic insult, Augustus A. White, M.D., a prominent orthopedist, says that a routine set of spinal x-rays in a young woman has a radiation effect on her ovaries equivalent to chest x-rays administered daily for sixty days [263:54].

Spinography, which is still done by about 20 percent of chiropractors, is not the only source of unnecessary radiation of chiropractic patients. Many chiropractors use smaller, regional x-rays inappropriately. Even the judge in the lawsuit against the AMA stated that the chiropractors take too many x-rays (see Chapter 11). ACA members who responded to a recent survey reported that 96.3 percent of their new patients and 80 percent of their continuing patients were x-rayed [193].

Poor Advice about Immunization

Many chiropractors advise against immunization. In 1992, 37 percent of 178 chiropractors who responded to a survey agreed that "there is no scientific proof that immunization prevents infectious disease" and 23 percent said they were uncertain. Among the "unproven" group, 24 percent were ACA members and 65 percent were ICA members. Twenty-seven percent of the respondents said their own families had not been immunized [55].

The ACA and ICA both oppose compulsory immunization. In 1993, the ACA House of Delegates recognized immunizations as a "cost effective and . . . practical public health measure." The ICA does not acknowledge benefit and even sells a book called *Vaccination: 100 Years of Orthodox Research Shows that Vaccines Represent a Medical Assault on the Immune System*, which contends that vaccines are ineffective and dangerous.

Chiropractors staunchly opposed the use of the polio vaccine in the 1950s, and many still support that opposition, saying that the incidence of polio is cyclical and would have declined without any vaccination program. The fact is that since the vaccine's introduction, the incidence of polio has become extremely *non*cyclical. The present rate of polio is less than one hundredth its lowest level before oral immunization programs began, and public health officials have predicted worldwide eradication by the year 2000. This is one of the most dramatic success stories in the history of medical science's struggle to reduce suffering and early death. The same could be said of the vaccination program that rid the world of smallpox, a once prevalent deadly disease. Chiropractors claim that somehow this would have happened anyway. That simply is untrue.

In addition to denying the benefits, immunization opponents also magnify the risks. A small percentage of children given shots to prevent diphtheria, tetanus, pertussis (whooping cough), and measles will experience adverse effects—most of them trivial. However, the benefits of these shots vastly outweigh the improbable harm. Where immunization programs are lacking, preventable diseases continue to cause death and disability despite improved public hygiene. Several states that had belonged to the Soviet Union, for example, are experiencing a diphtheria epidemic due to waning of their vaccination programs.

Chiropractic opposition to immunization appears to be based on a combination of philosophy and faulty reasoning. ICA past-president Fred H. Barge, D.C., has stated:

> I am a firm opponent of artificial immunization and the antiquated germ theory on which it is based. . . .
>
> Chiropractic philosophy states that natural immunity is to be favored over any attempt to artificially immunize the body, and chiropractic's approach to health augments the body's innate immunological capacity. [15]

This statement, in line with traditional chiropractic dogma, is not merely unsubstantiated. A recent study by chiropractors found that manipulative therapy produced no clinically significant effect on five types of lymphocytes that correlate with immune-system functioning [36].

Robert Anderson, M.D., D.C., believes that chiropractors "tend to evaluate all things medical in symbolic terms as hostile and harmful" [6]. In line with this, Craig E. Nelson, D.C., suggests that "it is precisely because opposing immunization sets chiropractic apart from medicine that makes this position so attractive to some chiropractors. . . . By opposing immunization, chiropractic ensures that it will not become assimilated into the health-care mainstream" [171]. Regardless of the reason, opposition to proven public health measures is irresponsible and can cause serious harm both to patients and to our society as a whole.

Financial Injury

Another risk common to chiropractic is that of "treatment" based on a diagnosis made with one of chiropractic's pseudoscientific tests. Such treatments, along with "preventive maintenance" adjustments, are useless and unethical. They are also expensive, because they usually involve a long series of "treatments" and may be administered throughout the duration of the patient's life. Harriet Cressman, mentioned in Chapter 5, paid a "discount" price of $10,000 in advance for "intensive care" after being told she would become a "helpless cripple" without it. Kurt Butler has described the case of a man whose bills from three chiropractors totalled even more:

The first did 185 spinal manipulations for alleged misaligned vertebrae over twenty months at a cost (to an insurance company through a workers' compensation program) of $4,000. The second chiropractor diagnosed hyperlordosis and rotational problems in the lower cervical and lumbar areas. He gave 207 treatments at a cost of $5,000. The third chiropractor diagnosed "chronic thoracic and lumbar instability" and gave 267 treatments for $18,000. Despite 650+ treatments costing about $27,000 over a ten-year period, the patient got steadily worse and never returned to work. These figures go up to 1987. As I write this in 1991, he continues to receive chiropractic treatments. [38:87]

Spinal Roulette?

In Russian roulette, the "player" spins the cylinder of a revolver loaded with one bullet, aims the gun at his head, and pulls the trigger. Few if any people play this "game" because the obvious risk far outweighs any possible benefit. The risk of being harmed and the probability of being helped by chiropractic treatment have not been measured. Thus the odds that an "average" chiropractor can provide you with safe, ethical, and effective treatment cannot be calculated.

15

Informed Consent
Is Needed

Accurate information is essential to make a free choice in any matter, but it is particularly important when it concerns health care. Yet few chiropractors provide patients with the information needed to make informed decisions about their care. Although full disclosure of risks is not legally required in every state, Peter J. Modde, D.C., and other chiropractic reformists insist that it is still a fiduciary duty—a matter of trust—which is a crucial part of the doctor-patient relationship. Patients entrust chiropractors with their health and pay them to act in their best interest. Rather than poisoning the therapeutic environment, as some would have us believe, full disclosure is simply an element of trustworthiness. It is unethical to neglect this duty for self-serving reasons.

Responsible chiropractors are concerned not only about the lack of informed consent, but also about the widespread use of misleading propaganda that leads to what could accurately be called "misinformed consent." Modde, among others, believes that "when a chiropractor distributes informational brochures which may tend to confuse or mislead a patient, he has created a situation in which the patient is so brainwashed that even a normally adequate oral warning might well be inadequate" [164:298]. Deception by chiropractors has been noted many times by independent investigators such as Consumers Union, the National Council Against Health Fraud, and the Ankerberg Theological Research Institute [8]. Charles E. DuVall, Jr., D.C., president of the National Association for Chiropractic Medicine, minces no words:

I think it is not only a moral and ethical obligation, but also a legal necessity to provide adequate explanation relative to the treatment or procedure so that the patient can truly make an informed consent—especially when there is *any* probability that the procedure/treatment may result in permanent impairment or death. This applies even though the probability of serious and/or adverse results is one in a million or even less.

If relevant information is withheld (a covert lie), or if false information is supplied (an overt lie), there is deception. Under such conditions, treatment is administered under false pretenses. Deceived patients are not able to choose freely. Only an informed choice is a free choice. Chiropractors who preempt their patients' ability to choose betray their trust and set them up for possible physical and psychological catastrophe.

The Legal Basis

The common-law basis of informed consent is embodied in the case of *Schloendorff* v. *Society of New York Hospital* (1914), in which the courts concluded: "Every human being of adult years and sound mind has a right to determine what shall be done with his own body." Most patients today want to share the responsibility for decisions about their health care. They are less inclined to accept authoritarian attitudes unquestioningly. They want to choose freely, which is possible only when they have adequate information.

Failure to obtain informed consent is a form of professional negligence. Basically, two standards for disclosure of information exist: (1) the medical community standard (physician-oriented standard), which reflects the prevailing practices of healthcare providers; and (2) the patient-need standard, which encompasses the information that reasonable patients would consider relevant to their decisions. Laws vary from state to state as to which standard prevails.

In 1986, David Chapman-Smith, an attorney who has represented and advised major chiropractic organizations, issued a report in which he stated: "I can think of few things that would hurt the interests of patients and the chiropractic profession as much as starting to warn patients of the risk of stroke" [41]. He suggested that chiropractors faced with a need to defend against "uninformed public comment" about the danger of neck manipulation keep their comments short and refer to "vertebral artery injury" rather than "the red flag word 'stroke.'" In 1994, however, he reported that "the strong trend towards patient rights in most countries suggests that there is a growing legal duty to disclose any known risk of serious harm, such as stroke or death, however remote" [42].

Essential Elements

Informed consent generally requires knowing the nature of procedures, the risks involved (both the likelihood and the severity), the potential benefits, and reasonable alternatives [39]. As applied to chiropractors:

- The complications of spinal manipulation can be quite severe. These include stroke, disc rupture, spinal cord damage, and paralysis. Lacking any systematic, reliable study of the frequency of complications, the likelihood is unknown and can only be guessed— a critical deficiency of chiropractic practice. In *Consent to Treatment: A Practical Guide*, attorney Fay A. Rozovsky advises that it is difficult to defend against a failure to obtain informed consent that is based on remoteness of the risk. She warns: "A defense relying on the definition of remote risks is more tenuous than one dependent on commonly known risks" [207:83]. In view of the limited benefits of spinal manipulative therapy, how many severe injuries must take place before patients should be warned about particular risks?

- The potential benefits of spinal manipulation are modest. Despite chiropractic's sweeping, grandiose claims, the scientifically supported benefits of spinal manipulation are primarily for low-back pain of mechanical origin. Many other chiropractic procedures have no scientific basis whatsoever.

- Alternatives to spinal manipulation are offered not only by various practitioners in the medical establishment, such as physical therapists or physiatrists, but also by chiropractors. Often there are safer options, such as exercises, moist heat, and massage. And some types of manipulation pose less risk than others. It stands to reason that manipulation may not be the most appropriate course, since 90 percent of back-pain problems resolve within two months with no treatment.

- Many chiropractors offer ill-informed, disparaging opinions about medical treatments.

Psychological Factors

Why is informed consent so important? One reason is that without it, people may well waste time and money on inappropriate or second-rate treatment for their problems. Another reason is that psychological damage occurs when a patient is deceived (either by a lack of pertinent information or by false information) and suffers a serious complication. Professional help may be needed to repair the damage.

An injured patient's distress will be intensified if, as often happens, the chiropractor disclaims responsibility for the complication. In my case, that is exactly what happened. The chiropractor not only denied wrongdoing but even rejected my eventual offer of forgiveness. After all—in his mind—he hadn't hurt me. I was to blame for what happened because my vertebrae didn't stay in place and chiropractors can do no wrong. He simply returned to business as usual.

I feel extremely angry about first being deceived and then being blamed for what happened. Can you understand how much difference it can make to someone injured by a procedure whether the risks were explained in advance? Knowing the risks provides an opportunity to decide whether they are worth taking. Being injured after a therapy is falsely portrayed as harmless is quite another matter. I was cheated out of the opportunity to make an informed choice. Others with similar experiences share the feeling that we were treated as expendable and sacrificed to maintain the lie that chiropractic is safe.

Support from Chiropractic Organizations

Chiropractic's major organizations recognize that practitioners have a duty to provide for informed consent. The American Chiropractic Association's 1994 policy statement says:

> Today, the standard by which the doctor is judged is that of "informed consent." By that is meant, to what degree has the patient been informed of all the potential consequences, dangers, and other factors, so that his consent is given with full knowledge of the inherent dangers to which he is exposed. [1]

The policy statement adds that "the public should be made aware that there are risks with manipulation."

The International Chiropractors Association has advised its members that: "'Informed consent' is a combination of (1) the legal duty or briefing of a patient as to the contemplated procedure; (2) forewarning the patient as to any possible adverse effects inherent in the procedure; and (3) the patient's acceptance of the risks involved." During the early 1980s, the ICA's legal counsel, James D. Harrison, wrote that "the stroke incident involving manipulation can no longer be considered a freak accident" [102] and that patients are legally entitled to information about the risk of stroke from neck manipulation [101].

The Mercy Guidelines (discussed below) advise:

> Patient consent to treatment is always necessary. It is often implied rather than expressed. However, where there is risk of significant harm from the treatment proposed, this risk must be disclosed, understood, and accepted by the patient. Such consent is required for ethical and legal reasons. [97]

The Canadian Chiropractic Association's clinical guidelines, which are similar but slightly more forthright, state:

> Chiropractors must disclose . . . any material risks including those that may be of a special or unusual nature. Even though a certain risk may be a very remote possibility, if it carries a risk of serious harm, it is a material risk and requires disclosure. [105:4]

The association's sample consent form, shown below, refers specifically to "stroke" and "serious neurological injury."

With all this organizational support (at least on paper) for informed consent, why do few chiropractors warn their patients that manipulation entails certain risks? There are probably three reasons. First, there is little or no legal penalty for not doing so. The issue won't arise unless a patient is severely injured and seeks damages for malpractice. Second, some chiropractors are concerned that informing patients about risks might induce them to forego "needed care." (This is why full information should be provided!) Third, and probably most important, few chiropractors believe that anything they do is dangerous.

Do Standards Exist?

In 1990, the Congress of Chiropractic State Organizations began organizing a group to prepare practice standards for the chiropractic profession. The resultant Commission for the Establishment of Guidelines for Chiropractic Quality Assurance and Practice was composed of thirty-five prominent chiropractors. After chapters were drafted and underwent review by outside consultants, the commission met for several days to reach a consensus on the many recommendations that had been proposed. The final

FORM OF CONSENT

Doctors of chiropractic, medical doctors, and physical therapists using manual therapy treatments for patients with neck problems such as yours are required to explain that there have been rare cases of injury to a vertebral artery as a result of treatment. Such an injury has been known to cause stroke, sometimes with serious neurological injury. The chances of this happening are extremely remote, approximately 1 per 1 million treatments.

Appropriate tests will be performed on you to help identify if you may be susceptible to that kind of injury. If you have any questions about this please do not hesitate to speak with Dr. Roe.

I have read and understood the above statement, accept the risk mentioned, and hereby consent to treatment.

Signed _____

Date   _____

Witness————————————————————————

Sample consent form published by the
Canadian Chiropractic Association in 1993.

report, generally referred to as "The Mercy Guidelines," was completed in 1992 and commercially published in 1993 as a 263-page book [97].

The published guidelines address more than three hundred aspects of the history and physical examination, diagnostic imaging, instrumentation, laboratory testing, record-keeping and patient consent, clinical impression, modes of care, frequency and duration of care, clinical reassessment, outcome assessment, collaborative care, contraindications and complications, preventive/maintenance care, public health, and professional development. Each clinical procedure was rated (in descending order of approval) as established, promising, equivocal, investigational, doubtful, or inappropriate. ("Equivocal" meant that a procedure's value "can neither be confirmed or denied.") The first three ratings were considered "positive" and appropriate for clinical use and insurance reimbursement. Procedural and administrative items were rated as necessary, recommended, discretionary, or unnecessary, while contraindications were rated as none, relative, relative to absolute, or absolute.

Although the Mercy Guidelines were a much-needed step in the right direction, they offer only modest guidance for providing informed consent. The report concludes:

> Numerous techniques and diagnostic methods . . . have been discussed in these guidelines which could not have been given a high rating due to the lack of research on the topic. Many of these techniques and methods are fairly widely practiced.

Under preventive/maintenance care, for example, the use of chiropractic adjustments was rated as "equivocal" because "the clinical experience of the profession developed over a period of nearly 100 years suggests . . . merit"—even though the Mercy conferees could cite no well designed study to support this assertion. (Perhaps we should ask how chiropractors can justify charging the American public hundreds of millions of dollars a year for "preventive" spinal adjustments that have not been proven to prevent anything.) The chapter on complications and contraindications concludes:

> At present, detailed systematic studies on this subject are lacking and the recommendations made are based on information from clinical reviews and case reports, as well as from expert opinion and consensus methods. One objective of this chapter is to encourage productive debate leading to firmer commitment on risk management protocols.
> . . . Research will be necessary to determine the true extent of the nature and occurrence of iatrogenic complications in chiropractic practice. The development of a central registry system capable of generating comprehensive research data would be valuable, and would facilitate the establishment of more detailed and refined guideline recommendations in the future.

Alarmed by the Mercy proceedings, the World Chiropractic Alliance reacted by holding a consensus conference and issuing a 123-page report called *Practice Guidelines for Straight Chiropractic*. Citing what it considers "overwhelming evidence," the report contends that "chiropractic care should begin at birth, when subluxation is likely to occur" and "be followed by a lifetime of continuing care." The report advises that, "in the interest of safety," straight chiropractors should "refrain from offering advice, diagnosis, prognosis, or treatment for non-chiropractic findings, while continuing to address the chiropractic needs of the patient." It recommends informing patients that "the professional practice objective of straight chiropractic is to correct vertebral subluxations . . . . regardless of the presence or absence of symptoms or disease" [200:30].

I interpret these words to mean that subluxation-based chiropractors should disclaim all responsibility for diagnosing anything but "subluxations." There is no mention of possible risks from manipulation. Do you think this is adequate or accurate information for making a wise decision?

Full Disclosure Is Needed

What would I consider adequate discussion of the risks? A Colorado chiropractor informs his patients that "manipulation is not a benign procedure and has been implicated in the aggravation of disc herniation or bony fractures, as well as the precipitation of vertebral basilar artery occlusion." This chiropractor deserves praise, but his message is still inadequate.

What would be adequate disclosure? I suggest:

> There is good scientific support for claims that spinal manipulative therapy can be effective in relieving some musculoskeletal pains of mechanical origin (not including pain from large ruptured discs, fractured bones, infections, or tumors). The known risks of manipulative therapy include stroke, disc rupture, fractured bones, paralysis, permanent joint damage, and soft tissue damage. The rates of these complications are probably small, but they have not been reliably determined.
>
> There are useful alternatives to spinal manipulation, and there are different types of manipulation, some of which are less likely to cause injury. The large majority of back problems do get better within two months of onset without treatment. Claims that spinal manipulation can remedy systemic diseases, boost immunity, improve general health, or prolong life, have neither scientific justification nor a plausible rationale.

Anything less, in my opinion, would constitute a form of "spinal roulette" played without the knowledge or consent of the patient.

16

Real Freedom of Choice

In an attempt to control rapidly rising costs, our health-care delivery system has been shifting toward managed-care programs (such as HMOs) in which primary physicians serve as gatekeepers to additional services. Under these programs, the patients' choice of providers is usually limited to those who have signed up with the plan. Managed-care companies try to select providers who are competent and do not perform unnecessary services.

The "Threat" of Managed Care

Traditional insurance plans permit patients to go directly to any practitioner they please. Managed-care plans provide unlimited access to one's primary physician, but specialized care must be authorized by that physician— usually a family practitioner. Chiropractors are worried that if they cannot be accessed directly, their income will suffer. Moreover, in communities where managed care predominates, nonparticipating chiropractors could lose their ability to earn a living. In 1993, the American Chiropractic Association included the following thoughts in somber testimony to President Clinton's task force on health-care reform:

> If we are to control costs, we must channel more Americans to primary care providers. Primary care identifies health problems early, before they become complicated and expensive to treat. It is preventative, emphasizing healthy life-style and nutritional habits. And it keeps people out of the expensive institutional settings.

185

These are all attributes of the practice of chiropractic and other non-MD health professions. I think the Task Force would be remiss if it did not take aggressive measures ensure that Americans enjoyed expanded access to all primary care providers, especially non-MD providers. . . .

First and foremost, government policies should provide an iron-clad guarantee that patients will have the freedom to choose their health care provider. Freedom of choice is fundamental to this country's traditions and should not be undermined in our health care system. In fact . . . . forty-one states have freedom-of-choice ["insurance equality"] laws guaranteeing access to doctors of chiropractic and many others ensure access to podiatrists, optometrists, psychologists and other licensed providers. . . .

Freedom-of-choice laws do not "mandate" coverage of new services. Quite to the contrary, they merely expand the pool of providers eligible to render care which is already covered under a health benefits plan. Such laws simply give patients the opportunity to choose any licensed provider to treat conditions or provide services authorized under the plan. In so doing, these laws expand the pool of providers without adding new services or costs. *The ACA would strongly recommend that any national health reform proposal include a guarantee of provider freedom-of-choice.* [10]

Is chiropractic care "preventative"? Should chiropractors be considered primary-care providers? Would including chiropractors in a national health-care plan cost nothing? Is the "freedom-of-choice" to which this testimony refers a legitimate concept? Let's examine these issues closely.

Preventive Care?

It would be interesting to know exactly what the ACA thinks chiropractors can prevent. The most common "preventive" measures chiropractors recommend are frequent spinal checkups and adjustments, which, as noted in Chapter 6, have not been demonstrated to prevent anything. Chiropractors have developed community and industrial programs that stress good posture and careful lifting to prevent back injuries. I am not able to determine whether these programs have practical value or merely promote chiropractic services. I can, however, tell you that the ACA's "public education" literature on these subjects has contained many statements like this:

Since it is impossible to restrain a child from participating in the numerous normal activities that may cause stress and strain, the correction of faulty body mechanics during the early stages is important. This is why doctors of chiropractic recommend that children have periodic spinal health examinations. . . .

Spinal disorders are often the result of twists, sudden turns, awkward lifts, and postural positions, and shocking body contact during play. If not corrected, spinal problems may lead to interference with normal nerve function and body mechanics causing or contributing to severe illness. [57]

Is there any published evidence that chiropractors are counseling patients effectively about good health habits? Have chiropractors demonstrated expertise by publishing the results of any program of smoking cessation, weight-control, or dietary modification? Have they contributed anything significant to the treatment of high blood pressure? Have they developed any interventions that can reduce the incidence of childhood illnesses or other infectious diseases? Have they promoted immunizations against childhood diseases or fluoridation to prevent tooth decay? Have they lobbied vigorously for laws that would lower the incidence of cigarette smoking or alcohol abuse? Do chiropractic organizations do anything that is not self-serving? As far as I can tell from reading their publications, the answer to each of these questions is either no or very little.

Primary-Care Practitioners?

Should chiropractors be designated as primary-care practitioners? Craig F. Nelson, D.C., a faculty member at Northwestern College of Chiropractic, recently answered this question in a chiropractic journal:

The phrase "chiropractors are primary-care physicians" has been spoken almost as a mantra without exploring the meaning of it. . . .

This 1992 booklet from the Foundation for Chiropractic Education and Research maintains that: (a) "chiropractic physicians address patient problems from the pediatric to the geriatric population"; (b) "chiropractic care is not restricted to any organ system, pathology or methodology"; and (c) chiropractors are able to coordinate patient care (including care provided by other specialists) and explain diagnosis and treatment to patients.

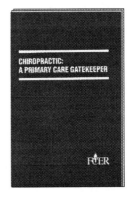

CHIROPRACTIC:
A PRIMARY CARE GATEKEEPER

FCER

> Chiropractic cannot have it all. We cannot claim to be generalists in the family practitioner mode and neuromusculoskeletal specialists and that we achieved all this in 4 years of professional training. It is an affront to common sense to suggest that this is possible. There is no evidence that chiropractors either function as, are trained as, are perceived by the public as, or are recognized by other professionals as primary care providers. . . .
>
> If we fail to define ourselves more coherently . . . . chiropractic risks becoming more peripheral and marginal than it is now. [168]

Extrapolating from two studies done by other chiropractic educators, Nelson estimated that during their four years of chiropractic training, students typically see approximately *two* new patients who come to the school clinic for something other than neuromusculoskeletal complaints.

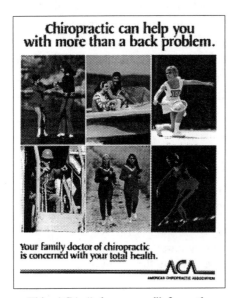

Chiropractic can help you with more than a back problem.

Your family doctor of chiropractic is concerned with your total health.
ACA
AMERICAN CHIROPRACTIC ASSOCIATION

This ACA "advocacy ad" from the mid-1980s alleges that chiropractic has a broad scope, but it does not delineate what chiropractors can treat. Specifying what they can actually treat would make it obvious that their scope is very narrow.

Whereas medical students examine *actual* patients throughout their clinical training, chiropractic students typically learn about pediatrics, obstetrics, infectious diseases, and other non-musculoskeletal problems from lectures, videotapes, and/or *simulated* patients (trained actors). Moreover, Nelson noted, "nearly all chiropractors go directly into practice following their 4 years of schooling, whereas nearly all medical doctors, including family practitioners, internists, etc., spend an additional 3–4 yr in residency training." Yet when an editor from *Consumer Reports* posing as a prospective patient asked 456 ACA members whether they offered "care for the whole family," most of the 274 who responded said they did so. Of these, the magazine reported, "nearly one-quarter . . . sent us material stating that spinal misalignments and 'interferences' with the nerves threaten overall health, and 35 percent implicated the spine in disorders of the body's organs" [47].

No Extra Cost?

Many chiropractors assert that they can function efficiently as primary-care providers by treating problems within their scope and referring the rest to other doctors. But it stands to reason that if common health problems lie outside of their scientifically supportable scope—as do the vast majority of complaints—seeing such patients will add unnecessary expense and delay appropriate care, even if proper referral takes place. And don't forget that some chiropractors try to sell every patient that walks through the door a lifetime program of "preventative maintenance." If an insurance plan permitted chiropractors to treat "subluxations" whenever and however long they please, do you think that would be inexpensive?

Freedom of Choice?

Is the "freedom" espoused by chiropractors a sound and democratic idea? William T. Jarvis, Ph.D., president of the National Council Against Health Fraud, Inc., thinks not. He regards it as nothing more than a ploy for weakening government protection against health fraud and quackery:

> Quackery's proponents invoke "health freedom," meaning that patients should be free to select any therapy they wish, and "medical freedom," meaning that practitioners should be able to prescribe any treatment that they and their patients agree is worth trying. The "health freedom" argument is a classic example of deception by misdirection. It focuses on the patient by offering to "give the dying man his last request." The reality is that patients may freely choose to do a variety of things. Patients may refuse treatments, swallow vitamins, eat apricot pits or the whole tree if they wish. However, [practitioners] may not sell their pet remedies in the marketplace if those remedies have not been proven safe and effective. The reason that patients clamor for dubious treatments is that they have been deceived into believing that these therapies offer hope. By focusing attention on the patients, the deceivers direct attention away from themselves. [121]

Remember that freedom does not operate in a vacuum. Insurance companies would like the freedom to choose what coverage they offer. Most would like to restrict their coverage to treatments that are reasonable and necessary. Chiropractic's "freedom-of-choice laws" (commonly referred to as insurance equality laws) restrict this freedom. And don't forget that someone has to pay for such treatments. "Insurance equality laws" can force employers and other policyholders to subsidize treatment they believe is inappropriate. If subscribers were asked whether their premiums (or taxes) should be raised to cover unproven "treatments," what do you think they would say?

Many chiropractors invoke the cry of "freedom of choice" to oppose immunization and fluoridation. The children who suffer from infections and tooth decay as a result certainly don't chose to do so.

The concept of "health freedom" did not originate with chiropractors. Historian James Harvey Young has noted that its use arose when our government began to rid the marketplace of dangerous and ineffective drugs:

> Before food and drug laws were enacted, quacks waived the banner of "freedom" to smear criticism aimed at them by physicians and pharmacists. . . . "Freedom" is certainly one of the most treasured words in the American lexicon. . . .
>
> Complex, modern, industrial, urbanized society, with its standards of medical judgment far more precise than in the nineteenth century, can not afford to let the nation's health concerns be governed by a distorted notion of that great symbol "freedom" which would return piratical anarchy to the realm of health. [272]

By providing this quote, I don't mean to imply that everything chiropractors do is quackery. But if you have read this book from the beginning, you will see that much of it deserves that label. True freedom requires a balance between freedom and regulation. We need laws that control deception and fraud in commercial transactions, particularly in matters that involve health and safety. If our government gives chiropractors complete freedom and financial support without responsibility or regulation, their quackery will keep expanding. Freedom also requires access to accurate information. Our society should strive to shine the light of science into every nook and cranny of the health-care industry. Only then will the public have real freedom of choice.

17

Can Chiropractic Be Reformed?

As chiropractic passes its hundred-year mark, where is it headed? Will it remain rooted to dogma? Will it become more scientific? Can its abuses be curbed? Meanwhile, what should consumers do? This chapter explores these questions.

Efforts at Reform

Breaking away from a cult in which one has become enmeshed is not easy. Many chiropractors were indoctrinated early in life through exposure to false beliefs held by their parents. At most chiropractic colleges, students who accept chiropractic dogma receive social reinforcement, while those who reject it face ostracism or even expulsion. Those who see the light after years of investment in training—or years of chiropractic practice—face a serious dilemma. Quitting may involve throwing away a large investment of time and money and, at least temporarily, giving up one's ability to earn a living. Staying put and working for reform can be equally difficult. Nonetheless, some do.

I use the term "reformists" to describe chiropractors who limit their practice to conservative treatment for musculoskeletal conditions and openly denounce chiropractic's subluxation theory, metaphysical notions, and unscientific procedures. Reformists post no charts relating "nerve interference" to diseases throughout the body. They distribute no brochures implying that spinal manipulation can treat disease. They only use diagnostic and treatment methods that have a scientifically plausible basis. Applied kinesiology and iridology, for example, are not among them. Reformists use x-rays conservatively, if at all. They inform prospective patients of the risks as well as the possible benefits of spinal manipulation. They regard overtreatment as unethical and an unnecessary risk. They support scientifically justified public health measures. They don't prescribe or sell vitamins or nutritional supplements in their offices. They do not tolerate the exploitative tactics promoted by practice-builders. Rather than denigrating the medical profession, reformists team up with medical doctors for their patients' welfare.

The first chiropractor to fit this description was probably Samuel Homola, D.C., who practices in Panama City, Florida. For more than thirty years, he has been urging chiropractors to become more scientific. His 1963 book, *Bonesetting, Chiropractic, and Cultism*, provides great insight into chiropractic's history and dogma.

The second reformist who came to light was Peter J. Modde, D.C., who practiced near Seattle, Washington. A 1964 graduate of Palmer College, he became president of his county chiropractic society and chairman of his state society's public relations committee. Somewhere along the line, however, he concluded that chiropractic theory was a delusional system and that chiropractors were not adequately trained in diagnosis. He began limiting his practice to physical therapy of patients that had been evaluated by medical doctors. He also persuaded medical doctors in Seattle to offer a special three-hundred-hour course in diagnosis. When his fellow chiropractors rejected this idea, he became thoroughly disillusioned, began publicizing his views, and offered expert testimony in malpractice cases. Prior to that time, suing a chiropractor was very difficult because it was almost impossible to find a chiropractor willing to testify against a colleague. Modde not only stepped on chiropractic toes by denouncing subluxation theory as a delusion, he also accused his colleagues of incompetence and threatened their financial well-being. For this, he was expelled from his state and national associations, his malpractice insurance was canceled, and an unsuccessful attempt was made to revoke his license [20]. He continued his reformist activities for about ten years but finally switched careers into real estate. His book, *Chiropractic Malpractice*, describes his experiences with more than a hundred cases.

Another reformist who left his mark was the late Charles E. DuVall, Sr., D.C., both of whose parents were medical doctors. (His father was also a chiropractor.) DuVall practiced in Akron, Ohio, for forty years and served on the insurance and industrial relations committees of both his state chiropractic society and the American Chiropractic Association. In 1981, he urged the ACA's board of governors to develop scope-and-conduct guidelines to counteract the problems he observed during his insurance work. When the board refused, he concluded that organized chiropractic would never reform itself from within. He and his son (Charles E. DuVall, Jr., D.C.) then wrote a scope-of-practice document, offered it to insurance companies, and began speaking publicly about chiropractic misconduct.

In 1984, hoping to steer chiropractic toward a sound scientific and ethical basis, the DuValls worked with Ronald L. Slaughter, D.C., of Houston, Texas, to form the National Association for Chiropractic Medicine (NACM), which soon affiliated with the National Council Against Health Fraud. To gain admission to NACM, applicants must sign a written pledge to "openly renounce the historical chiropractic philosophical concept that subluxation is the cause of disease," and to restrict their scope of practice to neuromusculoskeletal conditions of a nonsurgical nature. So far about three hundred chiropractors and chiropractic students have joined. Most are not politically involved, but some speak publicly about chiropractic's shortcomings, review cases for insurance companies, testify in malpractice cases, and/or assist investigative reporters. NACM also maintains a referral list for consumers who are seeking conservative chiropractic care. Chiropractic licensing boards have attempted to intimidate several NACM leaders by initiating spurious actions against them. In each case, however, the reformist fought back and won.

In 1994, Murray Katz, M.D.C.M., a Canadian physician, launched the Orthopractic Manipulation Society International (OMSI), an organization "dedicated to providing the public, fellow health professionals, and government with guidelines on the provision of safe and scientific manual, mobilization and manipulation therapy." This group, which is open to medical and osteopathic physicians, physiotherapists, and chiropractors, quickly attracted more than a thousand members. Its literature renounced "subluxation" theory and many of the dubious marketing tactics and therapies described in this book [127]. An American affiliate was also incorporated as an NACM subsidiary.

Organized chiropractic was enraged (and also frightened). The editor of *Dynamic Chiropractic* charged that "only a traitor would give up chiropractic to become an 'orthopractor'" [189]. One NACM member who spearheaded the orthopractic movement in his state even had his office raked with gunfire after he had received numerous telephone threats advising him to stop promoting the orthopractic concept. The International Chiropractors Association labeled orthopractic "a splinter concept of chiropractic contrary to the definitions of chiropractic embodied in state laws" and "an amalgamation of forces antagonistic to mainstream chiropractic . . . programmed by intent or misadventure to augment the efforts of political medicine" [114]. The Federation of State Licensing Boards adopted a position that the words "orthopractic" or "orthopractor" may be misleading, and several state licensing boards announced that users of these words would be subject to disciplinary action [45]. Various threats were also made against educators and researchers who had joined an orthopractic group. Feeling that the risks were too great, most chiropractors withdrew from the orthopractic groups. NACM, however, remains active.

Reform is also being promoted by a small cadre of chiropractic educators who hope that upgrading education and research will eventually upgrade the overall quality of chiropractic practice (see Chapter 13). Efforts are also being made to establish practice standards (see Chapter 15). It remains to be seen whether these will improve the behavior of the average chiropractor. NACM's leaders doubt that they will.

Why Comprehensive Reform Is Needed

Kurt Butler, health educator and author of *A Consumer's Guide to "Alternative" Medicine*, regards chiropractic as "a cancer of the health-care system." The National Council Against Health Fraud has said:

> A health-care delivery system as confused and poorly regulated as is chiropractic constitutes a major consumer health problem. . . . The chiropractic problem is so broad-based that every segment of the community involved with health care, scientifically, economically, legally or educationally, must inject itself into the chiropractic controversy. Only a comprehensive approach to a solution has any hope of succeeding. [196]

I agree with these assessments.

Public Education Is Needed

Chiropractic has received less critical attention than almost any other problem in our society. Although most people have a vague idea of what chiropractors do, few people—including health educators and health professionals—have detailed knowledge. The following measures would help.

• Health educators should make a concerted effort to obtain information about chiropractic's fallacies, convey this information to their students, and encourage textbook publishers to incorporate it into health-education textbooks. Guidance counselors should inform students about the true nature of chiropractic so they can choose their career direction wisely. Medical publishers should engage medical experts to improve the overall quality of chiropractic textbooks and should stop publishing texts that espouse "subluxation" theory.

• Physicians should inform their patients about chiropractic's shortcomings. However, they should keep in mind that not all chiropractors are alike. Those who are scientifically oriented should be supported and permitted to attend the continuing education activities of hospitals and other medical organizations. Physicians who encounter people seriously victimized by chiropractors should carefully document their stories and encourage them to contact the National Council Against Health Fraud's Task Force on Victim Redress. The American Medical Association should set up a standing committee to monitor and report on chiropractic and other "alternative" health-care methods.

Consumer Protection Should Be Increased

Chiropractors have been given the freedom to practice with little requirement that they do so in a scientifically responsible manner. Education alone cannot protect consumers or help people who do not realize that they are being deceived. The guiding principle should not be "freedom of choice" or "buyer beware" but consumer protection based on the rules of science. The following legislative measures would help.

• State chiropractic licensing laws should be brought in line with reality by (1) removing all mention of "subluxations," "spinal misalignments," "nerve energy," "nerve interference," and other nonscientific concepts; and (2) restricting chiropractors' scope of practice to neuromusculoskeletal problems.

• Laws should specify the procedures that chiropractors should *not* perform, such as colonics, herbology, hair analysis, cancer therapies, or any other unproven method unless working on a bona fide experimental project together with qualified medical researchers.

• Chiropractic use of x-rays—particularly the techniques that involve unnecessary radiation exposure, such as the full-spine x-ray—should be restricted. Chiropractors should be prohibited from taking x-ray pictures of persons under the age of eighteen, as was once done in New York State. The requirement that x-rays be taken in order to establish reimbursement under Medicare should be removed.

• Chiropractors should be prohibited from using the title "doctor" in any manner that does not make clear that they are chiropractors.

• "Insurance equality" laws should be repealed so that insurance companies are free to reject chiropractic care that is not cost-effective.

• Chiropractic training should be permitted in the same university systems that teach medical, dental, and other allied health professionals, so that instruction in basic sciences and training in diagnosis and patient screening can be brought up to the standards for other portal-of-entry health-care providers. The chiropractic degrees issued by these institutions could be designated "Doctor of Chiropractic Medicine (D.C.M.)" to distinguish them from current chiropractic diplomas. D.C.M.s should be permitted to utilize prescription drugs appropriate to the scope of their practices. Standards should be established so that holders of a D.C. degree can upgrade themselves to a D.C.M. degree. As an additional safeguard, the new programs should be accredited by the agency that evaluates the university's medical school rather than by the Council on Chiropractic Education. Western States Chiropractic College recently announced plans to start a D.C.M. program that includes training in a primary-care setting plus classes in diagnosis, drug therapy, and conservative management of common disorders. Although this is much less rigorous than a university-based program, it appears to be a step in the right direction.

• Chiropractic licensing boards should be given greater power to control chiropractic abuses. Funding should be increased and impartial individuals who are not chiropractors should be added to the boards.

Insurance Companies Should Become More Aggressive

Although most health-insurance companies are concerned about the cost of inappropriate chiropractic claims, few companies do much about them. The following actions can help.

• Insurance policies should limit coverage to services that are scientifically justifiable and to practitioners who provide appropriate documentation that establishes the diagnosis and justifies treatment. An effective program will probably require field visits to see whether billed services are actually being performed or whether, for example, dubious practices are being billed using standard codes. (An example would be billing an "electrodiagnostic" test as a routine office visit.)

• Managed-care programs should attempt to curtail coverage of inappropriate chiropractic treatment. Staff-model HMOs (where practitioners are employees) can accomplish this by hiring a scientifically oriented chiropractor to administer or supervise all chiropractic visits. Other programs can accomplish this through capitation (lump-sum payments regardless of the number of services used).

• The insurance industry should fund and cooperate with an independent commission that investigates health frauds and quackery and provides help in identifying and dealing with problem areas. The commission's findings should be published. An independent commission is necessary because sharing information with competitors could violate antitrust laws.

• When fraud or quackery is detected, it should be reported to licensing boards and law-enforcement agencies. This should be done routinely for all types of licensed health professionals, not just chiropractors.

Organized Chiropractic Should Promulgate Meaningful Standards

There is ample evidence that chiropractic education is defective and that unethical and unscientific practices are widespread among chiropractors. These changes are unlikely to be corrected unless chiropractic schools, licensing boards, and professional organizations establish and enforce meaningful standards. The Mercy Guidelines (see Chapter 15) were a good first step, but they are too vague and are not enforceable. Measures like the following are needed.

• The Council on Chiropractic Education (CCE) should upgrade its standards so that: (a) schools that promote subluxation theory or Palmerian metaphysical notions become ineligible for accreditation; and (b) students are adequately trained to determine whether patients have conditions that are outside the legitimate scope of chiropractic practice. This will require using some physicians as faculty members and ensuring that students have adequate exposure to patients with a broad range of health problems. Likewise, the National Board of Chiropractic Examiners should raise its testing standards to ensure that diagnostic competence is required for licensure.

• Chiropractic organizations should establish standards of practice and conduct that are clearly worded, consistent with scientific knowledge, and enforced. The process could begin by condemning the most egregious practices such as electrodiagnosis, surrogate testing, and the use of hair analysis as the basis for recommending dietary supplements. These procedures should be declared unethical, and chiropractic licensing boards should seek to revoke the licenses of anyone who uses them.

• Chiropractors and their organizations should abandon the nonsensical concept that "nerve compression" causes or is a major factor in disease. Reformist chiropractors consider this "the largest single step that chiropractors can make toward science" [69].

• Chiropractors and their organizations should join the rest of the scientific community in unequivocally endorsing immunization, fluoridation, and other proven public health measures.

• Chiropractors who support reform and are ashamed of what organized chiropractic has been doing should join NACM and work toward improving the situation.

How to Protect Yourself

Keep in mind that current laws offer more protection to health-care providers than to consumers; therefore choose your practitioners carefully—particularly if you wish to consult a chiropractor. Remember that although manipulative therapy has value in treating back pain and may relieve other musculoskeletal conditions, chiropractors are not the only source of manipulative therapy. If you do decide to visit a chiropractor, the following tips can help you avoid trouble.

• Never consult a chiropractor unless your problem has been diagnosed by a competent medical practitioner. Don't rely on a chiropractor for diagnosis. Although some chiropractors know enough to avoid diagnostic difficulty, there is no simple way for a consumer to determine who can do so. As an additional safeguard, ask any chiropractor who treats you to discuss your care with your medical doctor.

• Understand that some chiropractic treatments involve significant risk. Spinal manipulations involving sudden movements have greater potential for injury than more conservative types of therapy. Be aware that chiropractic neck manipulation involving extension and rotation can cause serious injuries. Even though the probability of stroke, paralysis, or other neurologic damage is small, such treatment cannot be justified on a benefit-risk basis.

• Do not submit to a full-spine x-ray by a chiropractor. This practice has doubtful diagnostic value and involves a large amount of radiation.

• Avoid chiropractors who advertise about "danger signals that indicate the need for chiropractic care," make claims about cures, try to get patients to sign contracts for lengthy treatment, promote regular "preventive" adjustments, use scare tactics, or disparage scientific medical care.

• Avoid chiropractors who "prescribe" dietary supplements, homeopathic remedies, or herbal products for the treatment of disease or who sell any of these products in their offices. For dietary advice, the best sources are physicians and registered dietitians.

• Avoid chiropractors who utilize acupuncture, Activator Methods, allergy testing, applied kinesiology, Bio Energetic Synchronization Technique (B.E.S.T.), chelation therapy, colonic irrigation, computerized "nutrient deficiency" testing, contact reflex analysis, cranial or craniosacral therapy, cytotoxic testing, electrodiagnostic testing, Essential Metabolics Analysis (EMA), full-spine x-rays, hair analysis, herbal crystallization analysis, iridology, laser acupuncture, leg-length testing, magnetic therapy, moire contourography, neural organization technique (NOT), Nutrabalance, NUTRI-SPEC, pendulum divination, preventive maintenance, reflexology, saliva testing, thermography, or a Toftness device.

• Urge your legislative representatives to introduce and/or support laws that provide greater consumer protection in health care, such as informed consent for chiropractic treatment.

• Choose your information sources wisely. The best sources about the chiropractic marketplace are the National Council Against Health Fraud (NCAHF), P.O. Box 1276, Loma Linda, CA 92354 (telephone: 909-824-4690) and Stephen Barrett, M.D., P.O. Box 1747, Allentown, PA 18105 (telephone: 610-437-1795). Barrett also chairs the Council's Task Force on Victim Redress, which assists people who feel they have been seriously harmed by any type of unscientific or quack practice. Of course, Victims of Chiropractic would be glad to help if you need information or support following a bad result from chiropractic. Its address is 1705 Liz Felty Lane, Bainbridge, GA 31717.

• Referral to a reliable chiropractor may be obtainable by sending a self-addressed, stamped envelope to the National Association for Chiropractic Medicine, 15427 Baybrook Street, Houston, TX 77062 (telephone: 713-280-8262). If no NACM member is available in your community, seek a scientifically oriented chiropractor—one who practices according to the principles listed in NCAHF's chiropractic position paper [196]. A free copy of the paper can be obtained by sending a stamped, self-addressed business-size envelope to NCAHF at the address above.

A Final Comment

I wrote this book as a way of constructively processing my anger and because I felt a social responsibility to do so. It reflects the most reliable information on the subject I could collect over the past few years. The book has been conscientiously and painstakingly researched and written. It is highly critical but proposes workable solutions for the problems described. It is not malicious in intent, but meant to help everyone, chiropractors included. I hope that chiropractors who read it will permit themselves to see the serious shortcomings of their profession. Doing this can be painful, but I hope that they will at least consider the possibility that they may have been deceived in some ways. Perhaps they will reflect on the origin of their profession or reconsider the importance of a scientific attitude and methodology in helping to ensure that their treatment is safe and effective. Only a scientific foundation can elicit the widespread acceptance and respect they desire.

For other readers, I hope the book's well-documented information will help you avoid the pitfalls of deception and provide the health smarts needed to receive high-quality health care. Perhaps some of you will care enough to share some of this valuable information with others at risk of being ensnared by quackery. A few of you may be inspired to investigate further and become involved in consumer-protection activities. Armed with the truth and motivated by compassion, a determined person can make a difference in this world.

Appendix A

Another Victim Speaks Out

Linda Rosa, R.N.

I remember a few things about being six. I remember adoring my first-grade teacher, Mrs. Pfeiffer, and delighting in my friend Ruthie's capacity to consume whole bottles of school paste. I also recall the day I stood before a strange, fat man with a bulbous, veiny nose who told me I would be hunchbacked and blind by the age of twelve.

My mother was—and is—a hypochondriac with an eighth-grade education. A tenant farmer's wife, she blamed poor health and the burden of childbearing for her lifelong unhappiness. Lacking confidence, she explained away her lost dreams with a multitude of ailments, the terrible symptoms of which I'm sure she sincerely felt and still feels. Her "doctor" for nearly twenty years was the late Dr. Lohr, a chiropractor who practiced in Rhinelander, some thirty miles from where we lived in northern Wisconsin.

Shortly after my mother started her own treatments, Lohr asked her to bring in other family members. A good thing, too, he told my mother after examining me. He could tell the instant I entered his office that I had serious problems. I would require vitamins and a minimum of one to three treatments weekly to stave off impending doom as a blind hunchback. And thus I was forced to begin what would be twelve horrific years as a chiropractic patient.

Lohr enthusiastically endorsed my mother's desire to avoid farm work, advising her to avoid any activity that might get her back "out of place" or "sublux" her vertebrae. My brother and I got the same orders (also no rough play or "sitting crooked"). This left my already overworked father

201

without support from his family, making him desperate, angry, and eventually impoverished. (Lohr gave my mother a supposedly *reduced* rate that actually was 25 percent more than the going rate for chiropractors at the time.) Bills for treatments, "pure" vitamins, and herbal laxatives ate up most of my father's income and, over the years, put us thousands of dollars into debt. My father's more emphatic protests were met by mother with theatrical suicide attempts. Ours was not a happy family.

From the beginning, I intensely disliked going to the chiropractor. What was there to like? There was the long car trip, missing school, hours of waiting in his office, the embarrassment of stripping down, the "liver pill treatment" and other such foolishness, and, of course, having my back "done." Even a kid could see through much of the trickery, and I resented being made part of it.

And then there was "The Machine." The Machine stood on a table in the main office. It had about a dozen dials on its face and a black hole about two inches wide near the top. Lohr turned the various dials with one hand while with the other rubbing a white washcloth dusted with talcum powder over a black square on the table. Connected to The Machine by wires were thick, black, plastic tiles which I was required to hold to my head, chest, and back. I never got an explanation of what any of this was supposed to do, though Lohr appeared satisfied with the dial settings only when the washcloth began squeaking.

After a while, an assistant would hook me up to another Machine in one of four small plywood booths, where I would sit holding the tiles with aching arms for fifteen to thirty minutes, incredibly bored as only a kid can be. After a time, The Machine was moved to the basement—more like a low, dank, and incredibly scary cave—the perfect antidote to boredom. My mother explained the move by saying that it was against the law to use The Machine. (Which, I must say, didn't exactly allay my fears.) I wondered at the time if its outlaw status had anything to do with a little girl I had played with for a time in the waiting room. She had been brought there to be cured of diabetes. Lohr had advised her mother to take her off insulin, lest she become addicted. The Machine and spinal adjustments would guarantee a complete recovery, he assured her. Unfortunately, she died before Lohr could cure her.

When I was very small, I worried that somber-faced Lohr could tell what I was thinking through The Machine. I thought he lectured me to be good and hit my back because he could tell how much I disliked him. After a while, I realized he wasn't picking up on thoughts or aches—or, for that matter, anything else from inside of me.

As a teenager, I overheard an assistant telling a patient that a saliva sample in The Machine's black hole would reveal to Lohr what ailed you—not only now, but in the future, as well—and, if you insisted, you could even learn the date of your death. My mother explained how The Machine measured the unique "electricity" of each organ. A certain reading indicated an organ's health. Poor readings could be adjusted by having The Machine restore optimum functioning of the organ. My mother said, "You could just sit there, and he'd tell you if your back hurt or your stomach hurt. Not everyone could use The Machine. Lohr tried to teach people, but only a few could ever work it. People got jealous of him, and they made it illegal." Yeah, sure.

Today I know that The Machine was an "electrodiagnostic" device, probably like one developed by Ruth Drown (the Drown Therapeutic Instrument), a chiropractor who got some of her ideas from Albert Abrams, a quack gadgeteer of seventy to eighty years ago. Abrams theorized that all parts of the body vibrate and emit electrical impulses of different frequencies, varying further if afflicted with disease. He called his studies "radionics." Drown died in 1965, while awaiting trial for fraud. She had sold a California Public Health Department undercover agent a Drown Therapeutic Instrument for $588, diagnosed the agent's children as coming down with mumps and chicken pox, and explained how to set the dials to cure the children at home. The specimens mailed to Drown for diagnosis were actually turkey, sheep, and pig blood placed on blotting paper.

After my sessions on The Machine came The Adjustment. I could see nothing as I lay on Lohr's adjustment table; my gown flopped open to expose my entire backside. I was cold and embarrassed. Lohr sat to my left, one hand wiggling my tailbone and the other rubbing areas along my spine so lightly that I wondered what possible effect he could expect on the bones below. Lohr used this time to lecture me on the value of Sunday School and obeying my mother. With my face wedged between two hard cushions, I mumbled assents.

And I tried to take my mind away, but I was never very good at that. I remained tense in anticipation of the two-fisted punch that he delivered to my spine at least once every week. It always came at an unexpected moment and sent me into something like spinal shock—dazed and stiffened as if treated to the business end of a cattle prod. I would have howled in pain, but for the air already having been knocked out of me.

Lohr had a penchant for gimmicks and gadgets (a common thing with chiropractors, I discovered later). In my teens, he started me on "liver pill treatments" (my name for it, though it was supposed to be diagnostic). Two major changes accompanied the liver pill. For one, my mother was brought in to observe my adjustments; and for another, Lohr now talked about what he was doing. It was Show Time. As I lay face-down on the table, Lohr placed what he called a "concentrated liver pill" on my back next to my spine. Thereafter, he had three seconds to get down to my feet where he needed to click my heels together three times. (I once remember hoping to myself I would end up in Oz—or even Kansas). Lohr prattled on to my mother how if the tablet lay next to a subluxation, one of my legs would immediately lengthen and the other shorten. This would only work, of course, if I was wearing shoes with leather soles. My mother could see it really happen, just as he said. At sixteen, I certainly knew better. I could easily feel Lohr pull and push on my legs as he knocked my heels together. By that time, Lohr must have felt confident that my mother would believe anything he fed her and nothing I said in protest. I was just "against him," like so many others.

Around this time my mother began dosing me with Lohr's imported herbal laxative (also said to be illegal). I don't know why it was thought necessary; I think I just had a cold at the time. I certainly hadn't been constipated, but that was to change. In short order, I became dependent on it; a dependency that was to last for four years. Considering that it caused me to faint nearly every morning, it's a wonder that my mother did not question its usefulness. It also caused considerable abdominal pain. Recently, I saw my mother taking a spoonful of the very same stuff. I asked if she didn't find it harsh and addictive. Quite annoyed, she replied, "No, it isn't! I ought to know; I've taken it every night for over twenty years!"

College enabled me to escape from this horror. Soon after I became a freshman at the University of Wisconsin in Madison, I made an appointment with an orthopedist to see what could be done about my chronic back pain. I mentioned that I had received chiropractic treatments for the previous twelve years and that the chiropractor had diagnosed "a bone missing" in my lower spine. (At the time, I thought Lohr might have been right at least about that—I mean, he took enough x-rays over the years.) The orthopedist misunderstood. He assumed that I had chosen to have Lohr's treatments, and he was enraged. Of course I would have pain if I let a chiropractor at my back. I deserved the pain. But when the orthopedist saw tears in my eyes, he softened somewhat and demonstrated an exercise that might help before showing me the door.

I wanted him to understand how much I hated being forced to endure the indignities of chiropractic care, but I fell silent, confused by his anger. I realized later that he must not have taken the time to calculate that I had been just a child, unable to refuse parental orders. How else could he have held me accountable?

But I left that doctor's office with more than an exercise. My eyes had been opened to the fact that my hated experiences were not part of a normal childhood. The cruelty I had suffered was just that, and not an accepted treatment for anything, as I had suspected, much less for the imaginary ailments with which I was "diagnosed." I confirmed then, and even more so after reading Ralph Lee Smith's book *At Your Own Risk,* the feeling that I had had all along—that Lohr was a quack, and that much of chiropractic was quackery. Lohr had not strayed from his chiropractic training but had built upon what he learned in school. He died, incidentally, a few months after I entered college.

It shouldn't take twelve years of methodical torture for a parent to see when a child is being abused. But my mother never has seen it, and that is a source of lingering bitterness by me. From an early age, I did what I could to rebel against going to the chiropractor—a healthy response for a child in those circumstances—but this ruined my relationship with my mother. To this day, she will not forgive me for not "believing in" chiropractors.

One cannot expect to put a child through that much during her formative years and not encounter some lasting effects. Still, considering the blows I took, not to mention supplements, laxatives, and x-rays, it is fortunate that I started out healthy and strong, with no real medical problems.

To keep from being taken more frequently to the chiropractor, I learned to hide any symptoms of real illness. Thus, no one knew I endured abdominal pain, back pain, sore throats, etc., during my teenage years. And during my first two years of college (before I could manage withdrawal from Lohr's laxative concoction), I even felt compelled to hide my fainting spells from my dormmates. My chiropractic-induced back pain, starting in my mid-teens, lasted for nearly six years after the treatments stopped. My university years were difficult; I had a hard time sitting in class or concentrating long on anything. Curious about science-based medical practice, I became a nurse. Recently, I began speaking out about pseudo-science and quackery (Therapeutic Touch, Healing Touch, and Rogerian Science) within my own profession.

In my case, chiropractic was a form of child abuse. For all its physical consequences, the greatest trauma was my exposure as a powerless child to frequent incidents filled with pain and hopeless terror.

Linda Rosa, R.N.
Loveland, Colorado

Appendix B

Glossary

Some terms in this glossary have more than one definition or are used ambiguously by chiropractors. The definitions below are consistent with the way these terms are used throughout this book and reflect what chiropractors usually mean.

ACA. Abbreviation for American Chiropractic Association, the largest chiropractic professional organization.

Accreditation. Certification by an accrediting organization that a facility meets standards established by an accrediting agency. Colleges and professional schools are accredited by agencies approved by the U.S. Secretary of Education (USOE) or the Council on Recognition of Postsecondary Accreditation (CORPA).

Activator Methods. Treatment system that uses leg-length testing to locate "spinal imbalances" and a spring-loaded mallet (Activator) to correct them.

Acute condition. Condition that has rapid onset and follows a short but relatively severe course.

Adjustment. Term most chiropractors prefer to describe their spinal manipulative treatment "because it signifies something more controlled, specific and skilled" [43].

"Alternative" health method. An unproven method that lacks a scientifically plausible rationale.

Amino acid analysis. Measurement of the quantities of individual amino acids in the urine or blood, a test that is falsely claimed to be valuable in assessing a patient's nutritional or metabolic state.

Applied kinesiology (AK). Pseudoscientific system of muscle-testing and therapy based on assertions that specific muscle weaknesses are signs of disease in body organs.

Asymptomatic. Free of symptoms.

Biomagnetic therapy. Pseudoscientific approach based on claims that abnormal organ function ("hypo" or "hyper") can be detected with "magnetic analysis" and remedied with magnetic and nutritional treatment.

C.A. Abbreviation for chiropractic assistant, a member of the chiropractor's office staff.

Cervical. Pertaining to the neck, e.g., cervical vertebrae.

CHIROLARS. A computerized database, available since 1990, containing citations and abstracts from chiropractic journals and other journals considered relevant to chiropractic.

Chronic condition. Problem that lasts for a long period of time or recurs frequently.

Clinical activities or subjects. Activities or subjects that involve patient care.

Consortium for Chiropractic Research (CCR). An organization of chiropractic colleges and agencies interested in pooling resources to sponsor research and conferences.

Contour analysis. Procedure in which an angled light is passed through a grid to the surface of the patient's body to produce a moire effect that is photographed. The resultant picture resembles a topographic map.

Contraindication. Reason that a diagnostic or therapeutic measure should not be used.

Controlled clinical trial. Research method in which people are assigned, under predetermined rules, to either an experimental group (which receives the treatment being tested) or a control group (which receives another treatment or a placebo). If subjects are randomly assigned, the result is a randomized clinical trial (RCT).

CORPA. Abbreviation for Council on Recognition of Postsecondary Accreditation (CORPA), formerly called Council on Postsecondary Accreditation (COPA).

Council for Chiropractic Education (CCE). The recognized accrediting agency for chiropractic schools.

Cranial. Pertaining to the skull, e.g., cranial bones.

Cranial techniques. A variety of techniques based on the incorrect notion that the flow of fluid surrounding the brain and spinal cord can be influenced by "realignment" of the bones of the skull; also called craniosacral therapy. This approach originated with osteopaths before they joined the medical mainstream.

Croup. An infection of the larynx (voice box) characterized by difficult and noisy breathing and a hoarse, brassy cough.

Cult. An unscientific system that involves devotion to a person, ideal, or philosophy. This description fits chiropractic's early years and is still applicable to subluxation-based chiropractic today.

D.C. Abbreviation for Doctor of Chiropractic.

D.O. Abbreviation for Doctor of Osteopathy. (See Osteopathic physician below.)

Dorsal vertebra. Another term for thoracic vertebra.

Double-blind study. An experiment in which neither the experimental subjects nor those responsible for the treatment or data collection know which subjects receive the treatment being tested and which receive something else (such as a placebo).

Dynamic thrust. A type of chiropractic manipulation that is sudden and forceful.

"Electrodiagnosis." Various tests in which a bogus device is used to detect "electromagnetic imbalances." (See Chapter 7.)

FDA. Abbreviation for the U.S. Food and Drug Administration, the agency responsible for regulating foods, drugs, cosmetics, and medical devices.

Foundation for Chiropractic Education and Research (FCER). ACA-affiliated organization that funds chiropractic research and distributes materials promoting chiropractic. Its publications include books and flyers that criticize antibiotic usage and recommend chiropractic treatment for childhood ear infections.

Foundation for the Advancement of Chiropractic Tenets and Science (FACTS). ICA-affiliated organization that funds research and distributes reports on the chiropractic marketplace.

Functional problem. Problem affecting the body's function but not its structure.

Hair analysis. Laboratory analysis of the mineral composition of the hair. The procedure is not a legitimate basis for prescribing nutritional supplements.

Health maintenance organization (HMO). Prepaid health plan in which patients receive care from designated providers who agree to abide by the plan's cost-control and quality-control standards.

Herbal crystallization analysis. Bogus diagnostic test performed by adding a solution of copper chloride to a dried specimen of the patient's saliva on a slide. The resultant crystal patterns are then matched to those of dried herbs to determine which "body systems" supposedly have problems and which herbs should be used to treat them.

Herniated disk ("ruptured disk"). Protrusion of the central gelatinous material of an intervertebral disk through its outer fibrous cover.

Homeopathy. Pseudoscience based on the notion that diseases can be healed by administering tiny amounts of substances that, in large amounts, would cause healthy people to develop symptoms like those of the ailment treated.

Hypertension. High blood pressure.

Iatrogenic disease (or symptom). Any complication induced in a patient by a physician's actions or therapy.

ICA. Abbreviation for International Chiropractors Association, the second largest chiropractic professional organization.

Immune system. The integrated system of organs, tissues, cells, and cell products (such as antibodies) responsible for recognizing and disposing of potentially harmful germs and undesirable substances that enter the body.

Informed consent. Permission given by a patient who has been fully apprised of the nature and risks of a proposed treatment.

Innate Intelligence. Chiropractic term for a "life force" or "vital force" that directs the functioning of every cell and organ in the body. Chiropractic's founder, D.D. Palmer, postulated that "subluxations" cause illness or prevent recovery by interfering with Innate Intelligence. Many chiropractors still hold such a belief.

"Insurance equality." Chiropractic term for laws that force insurance companies to include chiropractic treatment in their plans. Such laws typically require that chiropractic treatment be covered for any condition for which medical treatment is covered. As of mid-1995, forty-five states had "insurance equality" laws.

Intervertebral disks. Structures, between the vertebrae, that give the spine mechanical strength and cushion the bones. The disks are tough on the outside and jellylike on the inside.

Iridology. Pseudoscience based on the theory that most body abnormalities cause abnormal markings in the eye.

JACA. Recently adopted abbreviation for the *Journal of the American Chiropractic Association* (formerly the *ACA Journal of Chiropractic*).

JAMA. Abbreviation for the *Journal of the American Medical Association.*

JMPT. Abbreviation for the *Journal of Manipulative and Physiological Therapeutics,* the only chiropractic journal included in the *Index Medicus.*

Kyphosis. Abnormal rearward curvature of the spine resulting in protuberance of the upper back; hunchback.

Ligament. A sheet or band of tough, fibrous tissue that connects bones or cartilage at a joint or supports an organ.

Live cell analysis. Pseudodiagnostic procedure in which a blood sample is examined with a dark-field microscope to which a television monitor has been attached.

Lumbar. Pertaining to the structures in the rear of the body between the lowest ribs and the top of the pelvis, e.g., lumbar vertebrae.

Maintenance care. Care provided on a regular basis after a patient has regained function.

Malpractice. Failure of a professional to provide diagnostic or treatment services that meet prevailing standards of care.

Managed care. Health-care system (such as an HMO) that integrates the financing and delivery of services by using selected providers, utilization review, and financial incentives for members who use the providers and procedures authorized by the plan.

Manipulation. A forceful, high-velocity thrust that stretches a joint beyond its passive range of movement in order to increase its mobility. Manipulation is usually accompanied by an audible pop or click. Because of the speed involved, the patient does not have control and the potential for injury is greater than exists with mobilization.

Mercy Guidelines. Common name for the report issued following the consensus conference held at the Mercy Conference Center in Burlingame, California, on January 25–30, 1992.

Meridian therapy. Term that encompasses acupuncture, acupressure, and other techniques claimed to balance the flow of the body's "life force."

Metaphysics. The body of speculations, supernatural matters, and other abstract concepts that go beyond factual or scientific questions. Metaphysical systems cannot be tested by observation and are therefore akin to religion.

Mixer. Chiropractor who uses other modalities besides manual manipulation of the spine.

Mobilization. Low-velocity (non-thrust) movement(s), done with the goal of restoring mobility, in which the joint remains within its passive range of movement. The slow speed enables the patient to resist.

Moire contourographic analysis. See contour analysis.

Monocausal doctrine. Term to describe the notions of D.D. Palmer and B.J. Palmer that vertebral misalignments ("subluxations") are the cause of all (or almost all) disease.

Musculoskeletal. Relating to or involving bones, muscles, and/or their attachments to other body structures.

N.D. Abbreviation for Doctor of Naturopathy. (Naturopathy is a pseudoscience based on the belief that the basic cause of disease is violation of nature's laws.)

National Association for Chiropractic Medicine (NACM). Reformist organization whose members have renounced chiropractic dogma and denounced the unscientific methods used by many of their colleagues.

National Chiropractic Mutual Insurance Company (NCMIC). The largest chiropractic malpractice insurer in the United States.

Nerve root (spinal). One of the two nerve bundles emerging from the spinal cord that join to form a segmental spinal nerve.

Osteopathic physician. Graduate of an osteopathic medical school. Osteopathy was originally based on false beliefs but gradually abandoned them and incorporated the theories and practices of scientific medicine.

Otitis media. Inflammation of the middle ear.

Paraplegia. Complete paralysis of the lower half of the body, including both legs, usually caused by damage to the spinal cord.

Peer review. A formal review of clinical work, records, insurance claims, manuscripts, or research by colleagues who are assumed to have equal knowledge. The process is used by insurance companies, managed-care programs, scientific journals, research sponsors, and hospital committees.

Pharyngitis. Inflammation of the pharynx (throat).

Placebo effect. Favorable response to a treatment that does not result from pharmacological effect or other direct physical action.

Portal of entry. Term used to describe a health-care provider to whom patients have direct access (without referral from another provider).

Practice-builders. Individuals or organizations that teach chiropractors how to increase their income through marketing techniques, increased productivity, creative billing, and/or other activities. The term has a negative connotation because many practice-building consultants have recommended methods that are unethical.

"Preventive maintenance." Term chiropractors use to describe periodic spinal examinations and correction of "subluxations." The usual frequency is monthly or weekly.

Primary-care provider. Health-care professional who provides basic health services, manages routine health-care needs, and is usually the first contact when someone needs care.

Pseudoscience. A theory or methodology that is represented as scientific but has no basis in reality. Its proponents typically use scientific terminology and concoct evidence (or distort scientific findings) in support of their beliefs.

Quackery. Promotion of an unproven health product or service, usually for personal gain.

Quadriplegia. Paralysis of both arms and both legs.

Radiculitis. Inflammation or irritation of a spinal nerve near its origin.

Radiculopathy. General term for nerve-root disorders, most often caused by compression of the root. Pain, numbness, paresthesia (feelings of "pins and needles"), weakness, and decreased reflexes may occur in the distribution of nerves derived from the involved root.

Radiograph. Medical term for an image produced with x-rays.

RCT (randomized clinical trial). Study in which the patients are randomly assigned to the treatment and control groups.

Referred pain. Pain perceived at a location different from the actual source of the disturbance.

Reflexology. Pseudoscience based on the notion that pressing on the hands and feet can exert therapeutic effects throughout the body.

Reformist chiropractor. Term used in this book to describe chiropractors who limit their practice to conservative treatment for musculoskeletal conditions and have openly renounced chiropractic's subluxation theory and the unscientific procedures used by chiropractors.

Report of findings. A term used by practice-management consultants to describe the interchange in which the chiropractor presents his findings and treatment plan to the patient.

Risk factor. Factor that increases the probability that a health problem will occur.

Roentgenology. The study of diagnosis through the use of x-rays.

Sacral. Pertaining to the sacrum (the triangular bone at the bottom of the spinal column).

Sciatic nerve. A major nerve trunk that originates in the spine and runs through the pelvis and upper leg.

Scoliosis. Abnormal lateral (sideward) curvature of the spine.

Self-limiting illness. Ailment that usually subsides without treatment.

Simulated patient. An individual trained to play the role of a patient in a standardized manner.

SMT. Abbreviation for spinal manipulative therapy.

Spinograph. A 14- by 36-inch x-ray film of the entire spine, usually taken with the patient standing, that chiropractors use to look for "subluxations."

Spiritualism (or spiritism). The belief that the dead communicate with the living.

Straight chiropractor. Chiropractor whose practice is confined to manual manipulation of the spine—based on "subluxation" theory.

Straight leg raising. A test in which each hip is alternately flexed with the knee extended and the extent to which each leg can be raised is noted. The procedure stretches the sciatic nerve and can reproduce symptoms if a spinal nerve root problem exists.

Stroke. Sudden loss of brain function caused by blockage or rupture of a blood vessel to the brain. Also called cerebrovascular accident (CVA).

Subluxation. Medical term for partial dislocation of a bone. Chiropractors define "vertebral subluxation" in a multitude of ways (see Chapter 3).

"Super-straight" chiropractors. Chiropractors who believe that their treatment affects "Innate Intelligence." Their sole purpose is said to be locating and correcting vertebral subluxations, rather than diagnosing or treating disease.

Surrogate testing. Bogus diagnostic test in which one person undergoes muscle-testing in order to diagnose supposed "weaknesses," "allergies," or "imbalances" in another person held or touched by the first person.

Systemic disease. Diseases affecting the entire body or a particular body system rather than just a localized area.

Thermography. An imaging procedure that portrays variations in the heat emitted from body surfaces. The prevalent types are liquid crystal thermography and telethermography (to detect infrared radiation).

Third-party payer. Nonparticipant in the doctor-patient relationship (usually an insurance company or government agency) that pays for the care.

Thoracic. Pertaining to the chest, e.g., thoracic vertebrae.

Transient ischemic attack (TIA). Spell due to temporary drop in blood supply to the brain. The symptoms can include dizziness, nausea, vomiting, lack of balance, disturbed speech, double vision, difficulty swallowing, and/or headache.

USOE. Abbreviation for the U.S. Office of Education, formerly called the U.S. Department of Education.

Vascular. Pertaining to blood vessels.

Vertebra. Bony segment of the spine that encircles and helps protect the spinal cord and nerves. The plural of vertebra is vertebrae.

Viscera. The soft internal organs of the body, especially those contained within the abdomen and chest.

"Vital force." A term "alternative" practitioners use to describe a non-material force that enables the body to function and heal itself. (See Innate Intelligence.) The concept that living things function because of such a force is called *vitalism*.

Appendix C

References

1. ACA policy on informed consent. American Chiropractic Association/For Your Information, June 1994.
2. Action on chiropractic mocks accreditation. American Medical News, April 14, 1975.
3. AMA Department of Investigation. Educational background of chiropractic school faculties. JAMA 197:999–1005, 1966.
4. American Academy of Neurology, Therapeutics and Technology Assessment Subcommittee. Assessment: thermography in neurologic practice. Neurology 40:523–525, 1990.
5. Anderson FM. The steps to practice control. In Anderson FM et al. *Seven Steps to Chiropractic Success*. Carlsbad, CA: d'Carlin Publishing Co., 1985.
6. Anderson R. Chiropractors for and against vaccines. Medical Anthropology 12:169–186, 1990.
7. Andersson, GBJ et al. The intensity of work recovery in low-back pain. Spine 8:880–884, 1983.
8. Ankerberg J, Weldon J. *Can You Trust Your Doctor? The Complete Guide to New Age Medicine and Its Threat to Your Family*. Brentwood TN: Wolgemuth and Hyatt, 1991.
9. Are you puzzled by that pain? Arlington, VA: American Chiropractic Association, undated, circa 1993.
10. Askew R. Testimony of the American Chiropractic Association before the President's Task Force on National Health Care Reform, March 29, 1993.
11. Assendelft WJJ, Bouter LM. Does the goose really lay golden eggs? A methodological review of workmen's compensation studies. JMPT 16:161–168, 1993.

12. Babitsky S. Workers' compensation: rationing of chiropractic care? Journal of Clinical Chiropractic 1(2):8, 1991.
13. Bach M. *The Chiropractic Story*. Austell, GA: Si-Nel Publishing & Sales Co., 1968.
14. Badanes J. Is this a scam? Usenet posting, May 2, 1993.
15. Barge FH. Final thoughts: possibly true? Today's Chiropractic 22(4):105, 1993.
16. Barrett S. Commercial hair analysis: science or scam? JAMA 254:1041–1045, 1985.
17. Barrett S. A current fairy tale. Legal Aspects of Medical Practice, February 1979, p. 10.
18. Barrett S. How five chiropractors diagnosed a healthy child. Pediatric Management 4(11):31, 1993.
19. Barrett S. Should chiropractors treat children? Priorities 5(4):31–33, 1993.
20. Barrett S. The spine salesmen. In Barrett S (ed). *The New Health Robbers*. Philadelphia: George F. Stickley Company, 1980.
21. Barrett S. The spine salesmen. In Barrett S, Jarvis WT (eds). *The Health Robbers: A Close Look at Quackery in America*. Amherst, NY: Prometheus Books, 1993.
22. Barrett S. The spine salesmen. In Barrett S, Knight G (eds). *The Health Robbers: How to Protect Your Money and Your Life*. Philadelphia: George F. Stickley Company, 1976.
23. Barrett S. Views of a chiropractic critic: your real enemy is yourself. ACA Journal of Chiropractic 27(11):61–64, 1990.
24. Barrett S et al. Chiropractic: still not recommended. In Barrett S et al. *Health Schemes, Scams, and Frauds*. Mount Vernon, NY: Consumer Reports Books, 1990.
25. Barrett S, Herbert V. *The Vitamin Pushers: How the "Health Food" Industry Is Selling America a Bill of Goods*. Amherst, NY: Prometheus Books, 1994.
26. Barrett WP. The land of bombardment. Forbes, February 1, 1993, pp. 80–81.
27. Bauman N. Chiropractors: can't get no respect! (Or can they?). Insurance Settlements Journal, Spring:12–23, 1991.
28. Beck BL. Magnetic healing, spiritualism, and chiropractic: the union of methodologies. Chiropractic History 11(2):11–16, 1991.
29. Beecher HK. The powerful placebo. JAMA 159:1602–1606, 1955.
30. Beecher HK. Surgery as placebo: a quantitative study of bias. JAMA 176:1102–1107, 1961.
31. Beresford L. Is it time to back chiropractic? Business and Health, December 1991, pp. 51–56.
32. Bigos SJ. AHCPR low back guidelines and chiropractic care. Dynamic Chiropractic 13(10):41, 1995.
33. Bigos SJ, Bowyer O, Braen G et al. *Acute Low Back Pain Problems in Adults. Clinical Practice Guideline No. 14*. AHCPR Publication No. 95-0642. Rockville, MD: Agency for Health Care Policy & Research, December 1994.

34. Boshes LD. Vascular accidents associated with neck manipulation. JAMA 274:1602, 1959.
35. Brennan MJ. Perspectives on chiropractic education in medical literature. Chiropractic History 3:25–30, 1983.
36. Brennan PC at al. Lymphocyte profiles in patients with chronic low back pain enrolled in a clinical trial. JMPT 17:219–227, 1994.
37. Brown M. Chiro: How much healing? How much flim-flam? Davenport, IA: *Quad-City Times*, December 13, 1981.
38. Butler K. *A Consumer's Guide to "Alternative Medicine."* Amherst, NY: Prometheus Books, 1992.
39. Campbell LK, Ladenheim CJ, Sherman RP, Sportelli L. *Risk Management in Chiropractic.* Fincastle, VA: Health Services Publications, Ltd., 1990.
40. Carver W. *History of Chiropractic* . Unpublished manuscript, 1936. Cited in Beck BL (see above).
41. Chapman-Smith D. Cervical adjustment — the risk of vertebral artery injury. The Chiropractic Report, promotional issue, 1986.
42. Chapman-Smith D. Cervical manipulation and vertebral artery injury. The Chiropractic Report 8(3), 1994.
43. Chapman-Smith D. The chiropractic profession: myths & facts. Palmerton, PA: PracticeMakers Products, Inc., 1993.
44. Chiropractic information (press kit). Chandler, AZ: World Chiropractic Alliance, 1993.
45. Chiropractic licensing boards deem "orthopractic" misleading. Dynamic Chiropractic 12(24):1, 12, 1994.
46. *Chiropractic: State of the Art 1994–1995.* Arlington, VA: American Chiropractic Association, 1994.
47. Chiropractors. Consumer Reports 59:383–390, 1994.
48. Chiropractors: healers or quacks? Consumer Reports 40:542–548, 606–610, 1975.
49. Christenson MG, Morgan DRD. *Job Analysis of Chiropractic: A Report, Survey Analysis, and Summary of the Practice of Chiropractic within the United States.* Greeley, CO: National Board of Chiropractic Examiners, 1993.
50. Christiansen J, Gerow G. *Thermography.* Baltimore: Williams & Wilkins, 1990.
51. Cianculli AE. Chiropractic: A primary care gatekeeper. Arlington, VA: American Chiropractic Association Political Action Committee, 1992.
52. Cinque RC. Confessions of a chiropractic heretic. Unpublished manuscript, early 1990s.
53. Cohen WJ. *Independent Practitioners under Medicare: A Report to Congress.* Washington, DC: Department of Health, Education, and Welfare, 1968.
54. Coletti RJ. The manipulators. Florida Trend 35(2):32–36, 1992.
55. Colley F. Chiropractic perspectives on immunization. Dynamic Chiropractic 11(2):32,38, 1993.
56. Cooke P. The Crescent City cure. Hippocrates 2(6):61–70, 1988.

57. Correct posture aids in maintaining good health. Straighten Up & Enjoy Life (undated newspaper), p. 6. Arlington, VA: American Chiropractic Association, 1987.

58. Cotton P. AMA's Council on Scientific Affairs takes a fresh look at thermography. JAMA 267:1885–1887, 1992.

59. Council on Chiropractic Education. *Standards for Chiropractic Programs and Institutions.* Scottsdale, AZ: Council on Chiropractic Education, 1995.

60. Crelin ES. Chiropractic. In Stalker D, Glymour C (eds). *Examining Holistic Medicine.* Prometheus Books, Amherst, NY, 1989.

61. Crelin ES. A scientific test of the chiropractic theory: the first experimental study of the basis of the theory demonstrates that it is erroneous. American Scientist 61:574–580, 1973.

62. Deely JP. Report of director, health insurance, to the officers and delegates of the forty-fifth national convention of the National Association of Letter Carriers. August 1966, p. 53A.

63. DeRoeck RE. *The Confusion About Chiropractors.* Danbury, CT: Impulse Publishing, 1989.

64. Donkin S. Eating fit! Des Moines, IA: Foundation for Chiropractic Education and Research, 1995.

65. Division of Eligibility and Agency Evaluation, Bureau of Higher and Continuing Education: *Nationally Recognized Accrediting Agencies and Institutions: Criteria and Procedures for Listing by the U.S. Commissioner of Education and Current List.* Washington, DC: Department of Health, Education, and Welfare, March 1978.

66. Donahue JH. Are philosophers just scientists without data? Philosophical Constructs for the Chiropractic Profession 1(1):21–24, 1991.

67. Donahue JH. The trouble with Innate and the trouble that causes. Philosophical Constructs for the Chiropractic Profession 2(1):21–25, 1992

68. Dunn M. Inside chiropractic education: perspective of a student reformer. NCAHF Newsletter 11(5):3, 1988.

69. Dunn M, Slaughter RL, Edington K. Is there a chiropractic science? JMPT 13:412–417, 1990.

70. DuVall CE Jr et al. The effect of cervical spine extension rotation on vertebral artery flow as found using digital EEG measurements on patients prior to manual manipulation. Research Thesis, Lynn University, 1994.

71. Eisele JW, Reay DT. Deaths from coffee enemas. JAMA 244:1608–1609, 1980.

72. 11 common questions about chiropractic (pamphlet). Arlington, VA: International Chiropractors Association, undated, early 1990s.

73. Ferguson A, Wiese G. How many chiropractic schools? An analysis of institutions that offered the D.C. degree. Chiropractic History 8(1):27–36, 1988.

74. Fernandez PG. *1,000 & One Ways to Attract New Patients.* St. Petersburg, FL: Valkyrie Publishing House, Inc., 1981.

75. Ferreri CA. *N.O.T. Basic Procedures.* Brooklyn, NY: Ferreri Institute, 1991.
76. Fickel TE. An analysis of the carcinogenicity of full spine radiography. ACA Journal of Chiropractic 23(5):61–66, 1986.
77. Fickel TE. Organ-specific dosimetry in spinal radiography: an analysis of genetic and somatic effects. JMPT 11:3–9, 1988.
78. Fishbein M. *Fads and Quackery in Healing.* New York: Blue Ribbon Books, 1932.
79. Foods, drugs, or frauds? Consumer Reports 50:275–283, 1985.
80. Frumkin LR, Baloh RW. Wallenberg's syndrome following neck manipulation. Neurology 40:611–615, 1990.
81. Fultz O. Chiropractic: What can it do for you? American Health 11(3):41–43, 1992.
82. Gatterman MI. *Chiropractic Management of Spine Disorders.* Baltimore: Williams & Wilkins, 1990.
83. Gatterman MI. *Foundations of Chiropractic: Subluxation.* St. Louis: Mosby Year Book, 1995.
84. Gaucher-Peslherbe PL. *Chiropractic: Early Concepts in Their Historical Setting.* Lombard, IL: National College of Chiropractic, 1993.
85. Gerber JM. *Handbook of Preventive and Therapeutic Nutrition.* Gaithersburg, MD: Aspen Publishers, Inc., 1993.
86. Getzendanner S: Memorandum opinion and order in Wilk et al v. AMA et al. 671 F Supp 1465, U.S. District Court for the Northern District of Illinois, Eastern Division, September 25, 1987.
87. Gevitz N. *The D.O.'s: Osteopathic Medicine in America.* Baltimore: Johns Hopkins University Press, 1982.
88. Gibbons RW. Chiropractic history: lost, strayed or stolen. ACA Journal of Chiropractic 13(1):18–24, 1976.
89. Gillins P. Insurance fraud: a winnable war. Healthline 10:12–13, 16, 1991.
90. Gross HW et al. Chiropractic coverage under Medicare. Testimony submitted to the U.S. Senate Finance Committee. Allentown, PA: Lehigh Valley Committee Against Health Fraud, Inc., February 15, 1972.
91. Gurin J. Letter to William J. Laurenti, D.C., January 25, 1995. Published in Dynamic Chiropractic 13(5):38, 1995.
92. Guyatt G et al. Guidelines for the clinical and economic evaluation of health care technologies. Social Science and Medicine 22:393–408, 1986.
93. Haas M. The reliability of reliability. JMPT 14:199–208, 1991.
94. Haas M et al. Muscle testing response to provocative vertebral challenge and spinal manipulation: a randomized controlled trial of construct validity. JMPT 17:141–148, 1994.
95. Haldeman S. The importance of research in the principles and practice of chiropractic. Journal of the Canadian Chiropractic Association, October 1976, pp. 7–10.
96. Haldeman S (ed). *Principles and Practice of Chiropractic,* Second Edition. Norwalk, CT: Appleton & Lange, 1992.

97. Haldeman S, Chapman-Smith D, Petersen DM Jr (eds). *Guidelines for Chiropractic Quality Assurance and Practice Parameters.* Gaithersburg, MD: Aspen Publishers, Inc., 1993.
98. Hall H. An analysis of "The Effectiveness and Cost-Effectiveness of Chiropractic Management of Back Pain." Unpublished report, 1994.
99. Hanczaryk M. Getting to the top – and staying there. In Anderson FM et al. *Seven Steps to Chiropractic Success.* Carlsbad, CA: d'Carlin Publishing Co., 1985.
100. Haney DQ. Twist of the neck can cause stroke warn doctors. Associated Press news release, February 19, 1994.
101. Harrison JD. Informed consent: a growing obligation. ICA Malpractice Alert, February 1982.
102. Harrison JD. Strokes. ICA Malpractice Alert, November 1981.
103. Health policy paradox (editorial). The New York Times, November 18, 1972.
104. Hender H. Preface. In Palmer BJ. *The Bigness of the Fellow Within.* Davenport, IA: Palmer School of Chiropractic, 1949.
105. Henderson D et al. *Clinical Guidelines for Chiropractic Practice in Canada.* Toronto: Canadian Chiropractic Association, 1994.
106. Hoehler FK et al. Spinal manipulation for low-back pain. JAMA 245:1835–1838, 1981.
107. Homola S. *Bonesetting, Chiropractic, and Cultism.* Panama City, FL: Critique Books. 1963.
108. Homola S. Seeking a common denominator in the use of spinal manipulation. Chiropractic Technique 4:61–63, 1992.
109. Homola S. Sense & nonsense in chiropractic care of the back. Scholastic Coach and Athletic Director 64(8):32, 34, 36, 1995.
110. How DCs in the USA practice. *Dynamic Chiropractic* 6(17):3, 1988.
111. Howe CA. Chiropractic approaches to pregnancy and pediatric care. In Plaugher G, Lopes MA (eds). *Textbook of Clinical Chiropractic: A Specific Biomechanical Approach.* Baltimore: Williams & Wilkins, 1993.
112. Howe CA. Pediatric chiropractic education: a paradigm. The Markson Practice Management Quarterly 1(2):3, 1993.
113. Hutchinson MA. *Bobby and Sue Visit the Doctor of Chiropractic.* Des Moines, IA: American Chiropractic Association, 1969.
114. International Chiropractors Association. ICA board takes emphatic stand on "orthopractic" and "chiropractic medicine." Today's Chiropractic 24(2): 86–87, 1995.
115. Jackson R. *The Cervical Syndrome.* Springfield, IL: Charles C Thomas, 1966.
116. Jamison JR. Drugs in chiropractic clinical practice: contemplating the variables which influence utility. JMPT 14:255–261, 1991.
117. Jamison JR. *Health Promotion for Chiropractic Practice.* Gaithersburg, MD: Aspen Publishers, Inc., 1991.
118. Jarvis KB, Phillips RB, Morris EK. Cost per case comparison of back injury claims of chiropractic versus medical management for conditions with

identical diagnostic codes. Journal of Occupational Medicine 33:847–852, 1991.

119. Jarvis WT. Chiropractic: controversial health care. Ministry, May 1990, pp. 25–29.

120. Jarvis WT. Chiropractic: a skeptical view. The Skeptical Inquirer 12:47–55, 1987.

121. Jarvis WT. How quackery is promoted. In Barrett S, Cassileth BR. *Dubious Cancer Treatment.* Tampa, FL: American Cancer Society (Florida Division), 1991.

122. Jarvis WT. Quackery: a national scandal. Clinical Chemistry 38:1574–1586, 1992.

123. Jarvis WT, Barrett S. How quackery sells. In Barrett S, Jarvis WT (eds). *The Health Robbers: A Close Look at Quackery in America.* Amherst, NY: Prometheus Books, 1993.

124. Jensen B. *Iridology Simplified.* Escondido, CA: Iridologists International, 1980.

125. Johnson RM, Crelin ES et al. Some new observations on the functional anatomy of the lower cervical spine. Clinical Orthopedics 3:192–200, 1975.

126. Kassberg M. How chiropractors are manipulating your patients. Pediatric Management 4(11):23–34, 1993.

127. Katz M et al. Orthopractic Manipulation Society of North America (flyer). Beaconsfield, Quebec: Orthopractic Manipulation Society of North America, 1994.

128. Keating JC Jr. Beyond the theosophy of chiropractic. JMPT 12:147–150, 1989.

129. Keating JC Jr. Slow progress. Dynamic Chiropractic 11(23):44, 1993.

130. Keating JC Jr. *Toward a Philosophy of the Science of Chiropractic.* Stockton, CA: Stockton Foundation for Chiropractic Research, 1992.

131. Keating JC Jr et al. Interexaminer reliability of eight evaluative dimensions of lumbar segmental abnormalities. JMPT 13:463–470, 1990.

132. Keating JC Jr et al. Journal of Manipulative & Physiological Therapeutics: a bibliographic analysis. JMPT 12:15–20, 1989.

133. Kenney JJ et al. Applied kinesiology unreliable for assessing nutrient status. Journal of the American Dietetic Association 88:698–704, 1988.

134. King FJ Jr. Ryan Itis: a homeopathic case study. Digest of Chiropractic Economics 34:46–47, June 1992.

135. King FJ Jr. Utilizing the homeopathic health appraisal questionnaire. The Chiropractic Journal 4(12):20,40, 1990.

136. Klein AC, Sobel D. *Backache Relief.* New York: Signet/New American Library, 1985.

137. Klinkoski B, Leboeuf C. A review of research papers published by the International College of Applied Kinesiology from 1981 to 1987. JMPT 13:190–194, 1990.

138. Knipschild P. Looking for gall bladder disease in the patient's iris. British Medical Journal 307:1578–1581, 1988.

139. Koes BW et al. Spinal manipulation and mobilisation for back and neck pain: a blinded review. British Medical Journal 303:1298–1303, 1991.

140. Kritz FL. What's covered: insurance companies still take a wary view of alternative therapies. Good Housekeeping, March 1994, p. 120.

141. Lamm LC, Wegner E, Collord D. Chiropractic scope of practice: what the law allows—update 1993. JMPT 18:16–20, 1995.

142. Lawrence KE, Painter SJ. *Chiropractic Patient Resource Manual.* Gaithersburg, MD: Aspen Publishers, Inc., 1993.

143. Leach RA. *The Chiropractic Theories: A Synopsis of Scientific Research.* Baltimore: Williams & Wilkins, 1986.

144. Lee KP, Carlini WG, McCormick GF, Albers GW. Neurologic complications following chiropractic manipulation: a survey of California neurologists. Neurology 45:1213–1215, 1995.

145. Lewit K. *Manipulative Therapy in Rehabilitation of the Locomotor System.* Boston: Butterworths, 1985.

146. Lewit K, Liebenson C. Palpation—problems and implications. JMPT 16:586–590, 1993.

147. Livingston MCP. Spinal manipulation causing injury. Clinical Orthopedics 81:82–86, 1971.

148. Localio AR et al. Relation between malpractice claims and adverse events due to negligence. New England Journal of Medicine 325:245–251, 1991.

149. Logan HB. *Textbook of Logan Basic Methods.* St. Louis: Logan College of Chiropractic, 1950.

150. Lowell J. Bilateral Nasal Specific. NCAHF Newsletter 8(1):2, 1985.

151. Lowell J. Live cell analysis: high-tech hokum. Nutrition Forum 3:81–85, 1986.

152. Lowry F. Orthopedists have bone to pick with economist over report on chiropractic. Canadian Medical Association Journal 150:1878–1881, 1994.

153. Lund SL. The most effective way to increase patient retention. Purpose Newsletter, Issue 3, 1991.

154. Lyons RD. 7 years of lobbying finally brings chiropractic under umbrella of medicine. The New York Times, November 19, 1972.

155. Maisel AQ. Can chiropractic cure? Hygeia 24:262–263, 1946.

156. Manga P et al. *The Effectiveness and Cost-Effectiveness of Chiropractic Management of Low-Back Pain.* Richmond Hill, Ontario, Canada: Kenelworth Publishing, 1993.

157. Mannello DM. Leg length inequality. JMPT 15:576–587, 1992.

158. Mas JL et al. Dissecting aneurysm of the vertebral artery and cervical manipulation: a case report with autopsy. Neurology 39:512–515, 1989.

159. Mas JL et al. Extracranial vertebral artery dissections: a review of 13 cases. Stroke 18:1037–1047, 1987.

160. Maynard JE. *Healing Hands: The Story of the Palmer Family, Discoverers and Developers of Chiropractic.* Mobile, AL: Jonorm Publishing Company, 1959, 1977.

161. Meade TW et al. Low back pain of mechanical origin: randomized comparison of chiropractic and hospital outpatient treatment. British Medical Journal 300:1431–1437, 1990.

162. Meade TW, Frank AO. Chiropractors and low back pain. Lancet 336:572, 1990.

163. Meyers AR. "Lumping it": the hidden denominator of the medical malpractice crisis. American Journal of Public Health 77:1544–1548, 1987.

164. Modde PJ. *Chiropractic Malpractice*. Delmar, CA: Hanrow Press, 1985.

165. Modde PJ. Malpractice is an inevitable result of chiropractic philosophy and training. Legal Aspects of Medical Practice, February 1979, pp. 20–23.

166. Moore JS. *Chiropractic in America*. Baltimore: Johns Hopkins University Press, 1993.

167. Moran WC et al. *Inspection of Chiropractic Services Under Medicare*. Chicago: OIG Office of Analysis & Inspections, 1986.

168. Nelson CF. Chiropractic scope of practice. JMPT 16:488–497, 1993.

169. Nelson CF. The cognitive roots of chiropractic theories and techniques. Journal of Chiropractic Humanities 1:42–55, 1993.

170. Nelson CF. Letter to the editor. JMPT 16:281–282, 1993.

171. Nelson CF. Why chiropractors should embrace immunization. ACA Journal of Chiropractic 30(5):79–85, 1993.

172. Nickerson HJ et al. Chiropractic manipulation in children. The Journal of Pediatrics 121:172, 1992.

173. Office of Technology Assessment. *Assessing the Efficacy and Safety of Medical Technologies* (SUDOC No. 052-003-00593-0). Washington, DC: Government Printing Office, 1978.

174. Office of Technology Assessment. *The Quality of Medical Care: Information for Consumers* (SUDOC No. Y3.T22/2:2M 46/12). Washington, DC: Government Printing Office, 1988.

175. Ostling RN, Blackman A. Is there a method to manipulation? TIME 138(12):60–61, 1991.

176. Ottina JR. Letter to Ernest B. Howard, M.D., received May 3, 1974.

177. Owens SE. Rebuttal: Crelin spine test not valid. ACA Journal of Chiropractic, Special Insert VIII:S54–64, April 1974.

178. Palmer BJ. *The Bigness of the Fellow Within*. Davenport, IA: Palmer School of Chiropractic, 1949.

179. Palmer BJ. *Fight to Climb*. Hammond, IN: W.B. Comkey Co., 1950. Republished, Kale Foundation, Spartanburg, SC, 1990.

180. Palmer BJ. *Selling Yourself*. Davenport, IA: Palmer College Press, 1921.

181. Palmer DD. *The Chiropractor's Adjuster: A Text-Book of the Science, Art and Philosophy of Chiropractic*. Portland, OR: Portland Printing House Company, 1910.

182. Palmer DD. The magnetic cure. Number 15, January 1896. Cited in Keating JC Jr. *Toward a Philosophy of the Science of Chiropractic*. Stockton, CA: Stockton Foundation for Chiropractic Research, 1992.

183. Panzer DM. The reliability of lumbar motion palpation. JMPT 15:518–524, 1992.

184. Parker JW. *Textbook of Office Procedure and Practice Building for the Chiropractic Profession,* Fourth Edition. Ft. Worth, TX: Parker Chiropractic Research Foundation, Inc., 1975.

185. Pedigo M et al. *International Chiropractors Association Practice Management Manual.* Washington, DC: International Chiropractors Association, 1986.

186. Peet JB. *Chiropractic & Pediatric & Prenatal Reference Manual,* Second Edition. Burlington, VT: The Baby Adjusters, 1992.

187. Peet PM. Foreword to Peet JB. *Chiropractic & Pediatric & Prenatal Reference Manual,* Second Edition. Burlington, VT: The Baby Adjusters, 1992.

188. Perdian TA. The light-force technique—a new perspective on the CVA scandal. The Digest of Chiropractic Economics, January/February 1993, pp. 30, 34.

189. Petersen DM Jr. The biggest mistake you could ever make! Dynamic Chiropractic 12(13):3, 1995.

190. Peterson D, Wiese G. *Chiropractic: An Illustrated History.* St. Louis: Mosby Year Book, 1995.

191. Pettersson H. *Activator Methods Chiropractic Technique*, College Edition. Phoenix, AZ: Activator Methods, Inc., 1988.

192. Phillips RB. Plain film radiology in chiropractic. JMPT 15:47–50, 1992.

193. Plamondon RL. Summary of 1994 ACA annual statistical study. Journal of the American Chiropractic Association 32(1):57–63, 1995.

194. Plaugher G, Lopes MA (eds). *Textbook of Clinical Chiropractic: A Specific Biomechanical Approach.* Baltimore: Williams & Wilkins, 1993.

195. Policy handbook & code of ethics. Arlington, VA: International Chiropractors Association, 1993.

196. Position paper on chiropractic. Loma Linda, CA: National Council Against Health Fraud, Inc., 1985.

197. Position paper on homeopathy. Loma Linda, CA: National Council Against Health Fraud, Inc., 1994.

198. A position statement: thermography. Park Ridge, IL: The Academy of Orthopedic Surgeons, 1991.

199. Powell FC, Hannigan WC, Olivero WC. A risk/benefit analysis of spinal manipulation therapy for relief of lumbar or cervical pain. Neurosurgery 33:73–79, 1993.

200. *Practice Guidelines for Straight Chiropractic.* Chandler, AZ: World Chiropractic Alliance, 1993.

201. Quigley WH. Chiropractic's monocausal theory of disease. ACA Journal of Chiropractic 18(6):52–60, 1981.

202. Quigley WH. The saga of the classroom building continues. Dynamic Chiropractic 6(12):24–25, 1988.

203. Ratliff C, Rogers S. A comparison of core curriculum courses common to chiropractic, medical, and osteopathic schools in Missouri. Journal of Chiropractic Education, December 1990, pp. 76–80.
204. Rehm WS. The end of an era: chiropractic's largest hospital is razed. Chiropractic History 13(2):24–25, 1993.
205. Root L. *No More Aching Back.* New York: Villard Books, 1990.
206. Rosenthal E. Back manipulation gains respectability. The New York Times, July 3, 1991, pp. C1, C9.
207. Rozovsky FA. *Consent to Treatment: A Practical Guide.* Boston: Little, Brown and Company, 1990.
208. Rueter FG et al. Radiography of the lumbosacral spine: characteristics of examinations performed in hospitals and other facilities. Radiology 185:43–46, 1992.
209. Sanders M. Take it from a D.C.: a lot of chiropractic is a sham. Medical Economics, September 17, 1990, pp. 31–39.
210. Sawyer CE. Nutritional disorders. In Lawrence SJ. *Fundamentals of Chiropractic Diagnosis and Management.* Baltimore: Williams & Wilkins, 1991, pp. 531–585.
211. Schafer RC (ed). *Basic Chiropractic Procedural Manual,* Fourth Edition. Arlington, VA: American Chiropractic Association, 1984. (Second and third editions were published in 1977 and 1980.)
212. Schafer RC (ed). *Basic Principles of Chiropractic.* Arlington, VA: American Chiropractic Association, 1990.
213. Schafer RC. *Developing a Chiropractic Practice: An Introduction to Tactical Chiropractic Economics.* Arlington, VA: American Chiropractic Association, 1984.
214. Schafer RC. The imbroglio of the professional greyhound. Dynamic Chiropractic 9(17):10, 1991.
215. Schneider M. Another look at preventive maintenance. Dynamic Chiropractic 13(8):20, 25, 1995.
216. Seminars of the Parker School for Professional Success. Fort Worth, TX: Parker Chiropractic Research Foundation, 1985, pp. 7, 39.
217. Shafrir Y, Kaufman BA. Quadriplegia after chiropractic manipulation in an infant with congenital torticollis caused by a spinal cord astrocytoma. The Journal of Pediatrics 120:266–269, 1992.
218. Shahid TS et al. *CHAMPUS Chiropractic Demonstration.* Aurora, CO: Department of Defense, 1993.
219. Shekelle PG. Letter to George Magner, September 19, 1994.
220. Shekelle PG. Note to Stephen Barrett, M.D., May 5, 1995.
221. Shekelle PG. RAND misquoted. ACA Journal of Chiropractic 30(7):59–63, 1993.
222. Shekelle PG. The RAND study: the appropriateness of spinal manipulation for low-back pain. Dynamic Chiropractic 9(21):1, 4, 39, 1991.
223. Shekelle PG, Adams AH, Chassin MR et al. *The Appropriateness of Spinal*

Manipulation for Low-Back Pain: Indications and Ratings by an All-Chiropractic Expert Panel. Santa Monica, CA: RAND, 1992.

224. Shekelle PG, Adams AH, Chassin MR et al. *The Appropriateness of Spinal Manipulation for Low-Back Pain: Indications and Ratings by a Multidisciplinary Expert Panel.* Santa Monica, CA: RAND, 1991.

225. Shekelle PG, Adams AH, Chassin MR et al. *The Appropriateness of Spinal Manipulation for Low-Back Pain: Project Overview and Literature Review.* Santa Monica, CA: RAND, 1991.

226. Shekelle PG, Brook RH. Editor's note. ACA Journal of Chiropractic 29(12):61, 1992.

227. Shekelle PG et al. Spinal manipulation for low-back pain. Annals of Internal Medicine 117:590–598, 1992.

228. Sherman MR et al. Pathogenesis of vertebral artery occlusion following cervical spine manipulation. Archives of Pathology and Laboratory Medicine 111:851–853, 1987.

229. Sherman RP, Ladenheim CJ. Truly informed consent: what MDs should reveal about alternatives to medical treatment. Journal of the American Chiropractic Association 32(6):45–47, 1995.

230. Simon A et al. An evaluation of iridology. JAMA 242:1385–1387, 1979.

231. Singer D. Effective patient retention. Purpose Newsletter, Issue 3, 1991.

232. Smith RL. *At Your Own Risk: The Case Against Chiropractic.* New York: Pocket Books, 1969.

233. Smith TK. Chiropractors seeking to expand practices take aim at children. The Wall Street Journal, March 18, 1993, pp. A1, A4.

234. Social Security Amendments of 1972 (Public Law 92–603), October 30, 1972, pp. 123–134.

235. Spector B et al. *Manual of Procedures for Moire Contourography.* Old Brookville, NY: New York Chiropractic College, 1979.

236. Sportelli L. *Introduction to Chiropractic: A Natural Method of Health Care,* Ninth Edition. Palmerton, PA: PracticeMakers Products, 1988.

237. Sportelli L. Marketing your practice in the 90's. Cassette tape #6. Palmerton, PA: PracticeMakers Products, Inc., 1992.

238. State of Wisconsin vs. S.R. Jansheski, December 1910.

239. Stierwalt DD. *Adjusting the Child.* Davenport, IA: No publisher specified, 1976.

240. Still AT. *Autobiography—With A History of the Discovery and Development of the Science of Osteopathy.* New York: Arno Press and the New York Times, reprinted 1972.

241. Strauss JB. *Refined by Fire: The Evolution of Straight Chiropractic.* Levittown, PA: Foundation for the Advancement of Straight Chiropractic, 1994.

242. Studies on chiropractic: a summary of published studies and official inquiries documenting the efficacy and appropriateness of chiropractic health care. Greeley, CO: National Board of Chiropractic Examiners, undated, circa 1993.

243. Sweere JJ (ed). *Chiropractic Family Practice: A Clinical Manual.* Gaithersburg, MD: Aspen Publishers, Inc., 1993.

244. Swenson RL. Pediatric disorders. In Lawrence SJ. *Fundamentals of Chiropractic Diagnosis and Management.* Baltimore: Williams & Wilkins, 1991, pp. 510–530.

245. Terrett AGJ, Kleynhans AM. Cerebrovascular complications of manipulation. In Haldeman S (ed). *Principles and Practice of Chiropractic*, Second Edition. East Norwalk, CT: Appleton and Lange, 1992.

246. Travel tips for good health. Arlington, VA: American Chiropractic Association, undated, circa 1993.

247. Triano JJ. Muscle strength testing as a diagnostic screen for supplemental nutrition therapy: a blind study. JMPT 5:179–182, 1982.

248. Turchin C. Improving relationships with the insurance industry. California Chiropractic Journal, November 1990, pp. 30–31.

249. Unorthodox "cure" for kids spawns lawsuits, outrage. San Francisco Examiner, March 6, 1988.

250. Utilization management applied to chiropractic area. Risk Management, August 1990, pp. 63–64.

251. Versendaal-Hoezee D, Versendaal DA. *Contact Reflex Analysis and Designed Clinical Nutrition.* Jenison, MI: Hoezee Marketing, 1993.

252. Vlasuk SL. Standards for thermography in chiropractic practice. In Vear HJ. *Chiropractic Standards of Practice and Quality of Care.*

253. Waddell G. A new clinical model for the treatment of low-back pain. Spine 12:632–644, 1987.

254. Walther DS. *Applied Kinesiology: Synopsis.* Pueblo, CO: Systems DC, 1988.

255. Wardwell WI. *Chiropractic: History and Evolution of a New Profession.* St. Louis: Mosby Year Book, 1992.

256. Wardwell WI. Chiropractors: evolution to acceptance. In Gevitz N (ed). *Other Healers: Unorthodox Medicine in America.* Baltimore: Johns Hopkins University Press, 1988.

257. Watt LH. *Handbook of Clinical Chiropractic.* Gaithersburg, MD: Aspen Publishers, Inc., 1992.

258. Weil A. *Health and Healing: Understanding Conventional and Alternative Medicine.* Boston, MA: Houghton Mifflin, 1983.

259. Weiss R. Bones of contention. Health 7(4):44–53, 1993.

260. Westbrooks B. The troubled legacy of Harvey Lillard: the black experience in chiropractic. Chiropractic History 2(1)46–53, 1982.

261. What we teach. The Chiropractic Journal 8(1):34–36, 1993.

262. When your health matters (flyer). Phoenix, AZ: Activator Methods, 1989.

263. White AA. *Your Aching Back: A Doctor's Guide to Relief.* New York: Fireside Books, 1990.

264. Why chiropractic is different (pamphlet). Spartanburg, SC: Sherman College of Straight Chiropractic, 1976.

265. Williams SE. *Chiropractic Science & Practice in the United States.* Arlington, VA: International Chiropractors Association, 1991.
266. Williams SE. Chiropractic's Machiavellian dilemma: it demands a change in direction now! Today's Chiropractic 21(1):7–9, 1992.
267. Williams SE. *Dynamic Essentials of the Chiropractic Principle, Practice and Procedure.* Austell, GA: undated, circa 1970.
268. Wilson GA. *Things You Should Know about Cancer.* Denver: Spears Chiropractic Hospital, 1956.
269. Worrall RS. Iridology: diagnosis or delusion? In Stalker D, Glymour C (eds). *Examining Holistic Medicine.* Amherst, NY: Prometheus Books, 1989.
270. Wyatt MA. Memo to John R. Proffitt, July 19, 1972.
271. Yochum TR, Rowe LJ. *Essentials of Skeletal Radiology.* Baltimore: Williams & Wilkins, 1987.
272. Young JH. Laetrile in historical perspective. In Markle GE, Petersen JC. *Politics, Science, and Cancer: The Laetrile Phenomenon.* Boulder, CO: Westview Press, Inc., 1980.

Index

Abrams, Albert, 203
ACA. *See* American Chiropractic
    Association
Accreditation, 23, 25, 49, 50–51, 207
    Council on Chiropractic Education
    (CCE), 25, 49, 51
Activator Methods, 56, 83–84, 87,
    116, 199, 207
Acupressure, 56
Acupuncture, 56
    meridians, 8, 87–88, 101
Adjustment, chiropractic, 207
Advertisements by chiropractors, 59,
    61, 62, 70, 90, 122
AHCPR guidelines, 39, 83, 143,
    150–152
Allergies, dubious tests for, 101, 110,
    199
"Alternative" health method, 207
American Academy of Chiropractic
    Pediatrics, 123
American Academy of Neurology,
    83, 166
American Academy of Orthopedic
    Surgeons, 83

American Chiropractic Association
    (ACA), 21, 35, 39, 51, 83, 141,
    154, 188, 193, 207
    advertisements in *Reader's Digest*,
    2, 42
    bumper sticker, 67
    and "chiropractic science," 158
    and colonic irrigation, 89–90
    diagnostic and treatment standards,
    81
    and free x-ray offers, 94–95
    and health-care reform, 185–186
    and informed consent, 180
    and monocausal doctrine, 31–32
    and nutrition, 110
    opposition to use of drugs, 97, 98
    pamphlets, 29, 63–64
    policies toward immunization, 174
    posters, 98, 114, 125
    and "preventive care," 77, 113,
    186–187
    promotion of AHCPR report, 151–
    152
    surveys by, 26–27, 32–33, 141,
    174

229